Fenbendazole & Ivermectin Protocols For Cancer

A Metabolic Framework For Repurposed Drugs & Integrative Therapy

Marsha Shepherd Whitt

Marsha Shepherd Whitt | No Bull Just Publishing

ISBN 978-1-966942-10-8

This workbook is provided for educational and informational purposes only and is not intended to diagnose, treat, cure, or prevent any disease. It does not replace professional medical advice. Always consult a qualified healthcare provider before making changes to your diet, lifestyle, or health practices.

Printed in the United States of America.

After you've read this book, I would so appreciate your taking a moment to leave an honest review, which helps others who are searching for this content more easily find it. Just scan the QR code below, or visit the link to be taken directly to the review page on Amazon.

SCAN ME

https://www.amazon.com/review/create-review/?channel=glance-detail&asin=1966942109&ie=UTF8

Dedication

To every person navigating the uncertainty of a cancer diagnosis, and to their loved ones who carry quiet strength in the background. This book is written in respect for your resilience and your right to informed, thoughtful care.

Contents

Introduction 11

Chapter 1 The History of Cancer Research, and The Landscape of Alternative and Adjunctive Cancer Therapies 15

Why Patients Look Beyond Conventional Cancer Care 16

Reflection Prompt 17

Otto Warburg 17

Young Hee Ko 18

The Rise of Repurposed Drugs: From Dewormers to Oncology 19

How Patient Forums Shape Protocol Adoption 21

Distinguishing Science from Hype: A Guide to Evaluating Claims 22

Chapter 2 Metabolic Therapies — Diet and Beyond 25

The Glucose-Ketone Index: Dr. Thomas Seyfried's Cancer Starvation Model 25

Reflection Exercise: Tracking Your Own Numbers 29

Implementing a Therapeutic Ketogenic Diet: Practical Steps and Pitfalls 30

Carnivore Diet for Cancer: When, Why, and How 33

Who benefits from carnivore? 35

Cancer and Carnivore 36

Chapter 3 Advanced Metabolic and Adjunctive Therapies 39

Press-Pulse Therapy: Theory and Application 39

Important Online Resource for Press Pulse Therapy 41

Interactive Exercise: Press-Pulse Journal 42

3-Bromopyruvate (3BP): Young Hee Ko's Innovation 42

The First Human Application of 3BP 43

Hyperbaric Oxygen Therapy (HBOT) 46

Chapter 4 Fenbendazole — Fact, Protocol, and Practical Use 51

What Is Fenbendazole? Origins and Human Adaptation 51

How Fenbendazole Works: Cancer Metabolism, Apoptosis, and Immune Effects 53

Documented Case Studies: Joe Tippens and Other Real-World Survivors 56

Breast Cancer 57

Prostate Cancer 58

Melanoma 59

Lung Cancer 62

Many Different Cancer Types 62

Step-by-Step Fenbendazole Dosing Protocols, Cycles, and "Stacking" 62

Interactive Tool: Daily Protocol Tracker 64

Chapter 5 Ivermectin — Mechanisms, Protocols, and Applications........ 65

Ivermectin's Anti-Cancer Mechanisms: Beyond Antiparasitics 65

Interactive: Quick "Ivermectin Mechanisms" Case Reflection 67

Human Dosing Protocols for Ivermectin: Safety and Scheduling......... 69

Practical Adherence Checklist 71

Chapter 6 Comparing and Combining Repurposed Drugs 73

Fenbendazole vs. Ivermectin: Synergy and Differences 73

Interactive: Protocol Reflection & Tracking Tool 77

Other Promising Repurposed Drugs 78

Case Study: Brain Cancer (Glioblastoma) 79

Case Study: Colon Cancer Stage IIIb: 80

Case Study: Pancreatic Cancer 1: 80

Case Study: Pancreatic Cancer 2: 81

Personalizing Your Protocol 84

Reflection Prompt: Building Your Stack 85

Chapter 7 Sourcing Repurposed Drugs Safely 89

Universal Principles for Vetting Suppliers 89
Understanding a COA 90
Supplier Due Diligence Checklist 91
Veterinary vs. Pharmaceutical-Grade Products 92
Quality indicators can help tip you off to a safer product. 93
Reputable Suppliers and Red Flags 94
Counterfeit products 94
Storage, Handling, and Shelf Life 96
Chapter 8 Integrative Oncology — Bridging Standard and Alternative Approaches 99
Defining Integrative Oncology 99
Interactive Reflection: 101
Real-World Synergy Examples 101
Working with Healthcare Teams 102
Patient navigators and advocates 104
Sample Scripts for Talking to Doctors 104
Chapter 9 Safety, Monitoring, and Legal Considerations 107
Side Effects, Contraindications, and Drug Interactions 107
Red Flag Symptom Checklist 108
Combining Repurposed Drugs with Chemotherapy or Immunotherapy 109
Monitoring for Success: Biomarkers, Imaging, and Symptom Tracking 110
When to Adjust or Discontinue a Protocol 111
Off-Label Legal Landscape 112
Veterinary Drug Use Patient Rights and Myths 113
Insurance, Documentation, and Protecting Treatment Choices 114
Chapter 10 Creating Your Personalized Protocol 117

Mapping Your Journey: Flowcharts and Decision Trees 117
Interactive Element: Protocol Mapping Exercise 118
Creating Your Supplement Stack: What to Include and Why 119
Avoiding Common Mistakes 121
Customizing by Cancer Type, Stage, and Treatment History 122
Decision Tree Protocol Mapping 125
Chapter 11 Mind-Body, Faith, and Emotional Resilience 133
Managing Scanxiety, Fear, and Information Overload 133
Interactive Reflection: Emotional Check-In Tool 134
Practical Stress-Reduction Tools 135
Grounding and Earthing: Science and Practice 136
Harnessing Faith and Spirituality 137
Building Your Support Network 138
Caregiver Strategies 140
Listening and Support 140
Self-Care and Boundaries 140
Communication and Appreciation 141
Chapter 12 Resources, Research, and Ongoing Learning 143
Understanding and Participating in Clinical Trials 143
Interactive Element: Clinical Trial Reflection Worksheet 145
Top Patient Forums, Advocacy Groups, and Continuing Education .. 146
Navigating Information and Staying Safe 148
How to Spot and Avoid Scams, Hype, and Outdated Protocols 149
Scam and Protocol Evaluation Checklist 150
Chapter 13 Rapid-Fire Questions: Clarity, Confidence, and Action 153
How do I know if a repurposed drug is right for me? 154
How do I avoid dangerous drug interactions? 154

Can I combine more than one repurposed drug at a time? 155
Is there any way to know if these protocols are working for me? 155
Where should I actually buy these drugs and supplements? 156
How do I calculate dosing for these medications? 156
What if I miss a dose? 157
Will insurance cover any of these therapies? 157
What do I do if my family or doctor thinks I'm making a mistake? ... 157
Can I change my protocol mid-stream if something isn't working? ... 158
How do I decide when enough is enough? 158
Are there any warning signs that mean I should stop immediately? ... 158
Do dietary changes really make much difference if I'm already on medication? 159
Should I avoid all carbs or go zero-carb/carnivore? 159
Is there any point using grounding/earthing as part of my wellness routine? 159
How can I protect myself from fake medicines online? 160
Do I need a prescription for these drugs? 160
What's the difference between "off-label" use and illegal use? 161
How frequently should I get labs done while on these protocols? 161
Can I travel while using alternative protocols? 161
Are there any supplements I should definitely avoid? 162
Do these protocols work for all cancer types? 162
What's the deal with "press-pulse" therapy? Is it worth trying? 162
When do I need professional help adjusting my protocol? 163
Interactive Tool: Personalized Protocol Audit 163
Is there anyone who shouldn't try these protocols? 164
Are there any clinical trials on these therapies? 164
If my cancer returns after remission, can I restart these protocols? 165

What should caregivers focus on most? ... 165
Do alternative protocols work right away? ... 165
Can I use these protocols alongside palliative/hospice care? ... 165
Should I share my protocol details online? ... 165
What do I say when friends offer unsolicited advice? ... 166
Can children/teens use these approaches too? ... 166
How do I keep hope alive during setbacks? ... 166
Does faith/spirituality really help healing outcomes? ... 166
Can I still work/socialize while using these protocols? ... 166
Who do I call if things spiral out of control emotionally? ... 167
Is there ever such thing as too much information? ... 167
Are there silver bullets—or just lots of little steps? ... 167
Will my story help someone else someday? ... 167
Conclusion ... 169
Resources ... 173
Tracking, Monitoring, and Planning ... 173
Sample COA ... 174
Patient Support Communities: ... 175
Smart Patients ... 175
Cancer Survivors Network (CSN) ... 175
Cancer Chat (Cancer Research UK) “Ask the Nurses” Forum ... 176
Facebook Groups & Private Social Media Communities ... 176
Joe Tippens’ News Interview ... 176
Reddit Sub-forums (Reddit r/cancer etc.) ... 177
Keto For Cancer Skool Group ... 177
Unnumbered Supporting References ... 180
Numbered References ... 184

Introduction

I never expected cancer to become such a central part of my family's story. My brother fought multiple myeloma for nearly seven years before he died in 2023. Watching someone you love slip away is its own kind of heartbreak. You see the pain, the exhaustion, the hope that flickers with each new treatment, and the frustration that comes when nothing seems to work. I felt helpless as I watched him try every option his doctors offered—chemotherapy, radiation, steroids that kept him from sleeping, pills with impossible names, pills so toxic you couldn't allow your bare skin to touch them—but his health kept fading. He trusted the 'experts.' He followed every instruction. Still, it wasn't enough.

Just when I thought our family had paid its dues, my sister and her husband were both diagnosed with cancer. Both, in the same week. The shock hit like a tidal wave. The fear came next, then the grief. I wanted to scream or run away, but neither would have helped. Instead, I kept searching for answers—real answers, not just the same old scripts.

This is where my journey began in earnest. My brother's battle and death, and then my sister and her husband's diagnoses, broke me open. I needed to know more. Why did some people get better while others didn't? Why did everyone act like the only hope was in a prescription pad or an IV drip? My grief and anger became a fuel that pushed me down a rabbit hole of research. I read studies, watched YouTubes, listened to stories from other families, and dug into the history of cancer research. I even earned a certification as a ketogenic nutrition consultant, because it quickly became clear that nutrition is ignored by most doctors (because it isn't taught in medical school), even though it holds so much power. I got more angry.

The deeper I went, the more I saw the holes in the system. Doctors, as caring as many are, mostly learn in schools where pharmaceutical companies fund and direct the content of the curriculum. They learn to treat symptoms with prescriptions, not address the root causes. They are rarely taught how food and lifestyle can change the course of disease. We see this everywhere. One story that sticks with me is the case of Charlie Abrahams, son of filmmaker Jim Abrahams. Charlie's epilepsy didn't stop, no matter how many pills or surgeries they tried—until he started a ketogenic diet at Johns Hopkins. His doctor knew about the diet but wanted to 'exhaust pharmaceutical options first.' Can you imagine? Charlie was just a little child, suffering, while the simplest solution was right there, patiently waiting in the wings. I got angrier.

This is not about demonizing doctors. Most are doing their best with the tools they've been given. The real problem is the system. It isn't set up to support anything outside of drugs and surgery. If you ask about nutrition, metabolic therapies, or even things like stress reduction or faith, you might be met with a shrug—or worse, a dismissive wave. I know how it feels to be desperate for something more, only to be told that hope doesn't exist outside the standard protocols. Still more anger.

That's why I wrote this book. I want to offer facts where there's confusion. I want to bring clarity where there's fear and overwhelm. My goal is to share what I've learned about alternative and adjunctive cancer therapies—from repurposed veterinary drugs like fenbendazole and ivermectin, to metabolic therapies like ketogenic and carnivore diets, to integrative treatments like 3BP (developed by Young Hee Ko) and hyperbaric oxygen. I'll walk you through the fascinating history of cancer research, from Otto Warburg's ideas about cancer as a metabolic disease, to the discovery of DNA by Watson and Crick, which changed the direction of cancer research for decades. For too long, we've tried to prove that cancer is a genetic disease, when in reality, the genetic mutations are mostly the <u>result</u> of cancer, <u>not the cause</u>.

This book will help you sort through the science and the stories. You'll find the facts about fenbendazole and ivermectin—how they work, what the evidence shows, and where to source them safely. I'll cover protocols for metabolic therapies, including how to measure your glucose and ketone ratio, and why this matters. I'll point you to resources that can assist you in doing this. You'll read about other adjunctive options like 3BP and hyperbaric oxygen, which are giving hope to people who want to use less chemo or radiation, or simply want to support their body's healing capacity in every way possible.

But health is never just about what you put in your body. True healing is also about the mind and spirit. Cancer brings fear, anxiety, and sadness. These emotions are real, and they can affect how the body responds to treatment. I want to show you ways to reduce stress, find hope, and stay grounded—even when the ground seems to shift every day. Practices like grounding (earthing), prayer or faith, and building emotional resilience matter more than most people realize. Your mind, body, and spirit are connected, and all deserve care.

I know you need clear, actionable information. This book will give you practical protocols, sourcing tips for safe veterinary drugs, guidance on how to calculate human dosages, safety checklists, and stories from real people who have walked this road. You won't just read theory—you'll get step-by-step tools to use right now, along with the transparency to know what is proven, what is promising, and what is still uncertain.

I promise to keep everything rooted in the latest research and real-world experience. If something is not yet fully proven, I'll say so. If it's promising, I'll explain why. My hope is that you'll feel empowered, not overwhelmed, as you read these pages.

If you're reading this, you're already asking questions. You're already searching for hope. I want you to know you're not alone. My family's story is woven into every chapter. I invite you to use this book as a roadmap, a guide, and a companion as you explore new options for healing. Take what serves you. Share it with those you love. Let's walk this new path together.

Chapter 1
The History of Cancer Research, and The Landscape of Alternative and Adjunctive Cancer Therapies

Sitting in a waiting room, clutching a list of questions for your oncologist, it's hard to ignore the pressure in your chest. A woman in her fifties quietly admitted, "I feel like my entire life is now measured in appointments and medication doses." That sense of being swept along by forces beyond your control is all too common. If that's where you find yourself, know you're not alone. Many in this situation begin to look past traditional treatments. Something within just can't accept that "this is the only way." A headline about a new therapy, a survivor's story, or the persistent hope that more must be possible—all may prompt a search for alternatives.

Why Patients Look Beyond Conventional Cancer Care

Most people don't turn to alternatives because they distrust doctors or oppose science. Rather, frustration and exhaustion with the limits of standard treatments—chemo, radiation, surgery—lead them here. Sometimes those treatments help; sometimes, they don't, or the side effects become unbearable, erasing normalcy. Relief from pain, nausea, brain fog, and emotional strain often feels out of reach. A new kind of helplessness sets in when doctors say, "We've done all we can," or offer only to "watch and wait." You may hear about experimental treatments or clinical trials, only to find that you don't qualify. Insurance often doesn't cover promising new options. These moments can leave you feeling boxed in and powerless.

Conventional medicine often focuses on disease management, not whole-person healing. Doctors treat tumors, but not always the person suffering. This gap motivates many to seek protocols promising more control, fewer side effects, and renewed hope when it feels scarce. People search not just for a cure, but for dignity, agency, and meaning amidst chaos.

Those seeking alternative protocols want three things: clarity, empowerment, and relief. You want protocols explained simply, not in confusing jargon. You seek specific, actionable steps—not just vague advice. You want ways to feel better now, not at some distant future point. Authenticity and transparency matter. You want to know what works, what's safe, and where to find genuine guidance, not empty promises.

The emotions fueling this search are complex: fear of dying or suffering, anxiety about disappointing family, hope that sometimes feels risky, and occasional desperation. Success stories about nontraditional therapies inspire—yet can also cause anxiety about missing out or making the wrong choice.

Exploring beyond established care brings real risks that aren't often discussed. There's danger in buying drugs from online or veterinary sources without knowing how to check quality. Some people abandon proven treatments for unproven ones, sometimes risking their health. Many protocols have side effects or unknown interactions. Misinformation spreads rapidly, making it hard to separate fact from fiction and safe hope from false promises.

Reflection Prompt

Take a moment to note what first made you consider options beyond mainstream cancer care. Was it a conversation, experience, or something you read? Write about what you hope to find—and what you most want to avoid—as you navigate these choices.

Otto Warburg

If you start reading about cancer's roots online, you'll quickly bump into Otto Warburg's name. He was a German scientist who, about a century ago, asked a simple question: why do cancer cells act so differently from normal ones? Warburg discovered that cancer cells gobble up glucose at a rate far beyond healthy tissue, even when plenty of oxygen is around. This became known as the "Warburg Effect." Instead of using oxygen like healthy cells do in their mitochondria—the cell's power plants—cancer cells run on fermentable fuels—namely glucose (sugar) and glutamine—a much less efficient way to make energy. Warburg saw this strange behavior as a red flag, signaling broken mitochondria. He believed this metabolic dysfunction, not random gene mutations, was at the heart of cancer. While most of mainstream oncology shifted focus to genetics after Watson and Crick mapped DNA (their work stemming from the data of the uncredited Rosalind Franklin), Warburg's observations kept nagging at researchers who noticed that tumors often share this odd sugar addiction.

This metabolic viewpoint changes how you think about cancer. It suggests that cancer is less about a mysterious genetic code gone wrong and more about cells getting stuck in a primitive survival mode. Mitochondria struggle, normal cell communication breaks down, and energy production shifts to fermentation in a desperate effort to survive. The result? Cells that grow, divide, and spread out of control. For patients, this isn't just trivia—it means there are ways to target cancer that don't involve attacking DNA directly. You can influence the fuel supply and the cell's environment, not just its blueprint.

Young Hee Ko

Enter Dr. Young Hee Ko, a scientist whose work revived and modernized Warburg's ideas. In the early 2000s, she discovered that a molecule called 3-bromopyruvate (3BP) can enter cancer cells and block their unique way of burning fuel. Cancer cells use special "transporters" to suck in more glucose and similar molecules than healthy cells do. 3BP sneaks in through these same doors and shuts down the cell's energy machinery from within, while mostly sparing normal cells. Dr. Ko's research has shown promise in lab studies and compassionate-use cases, with the hope that 3BP could offer a new kind of targeted therapy—one that chokes off a tumor's energy supply at its source. She continues to build scientific evidence for 3BP as both a metabolic and immunological modulator[1], and has gained FDA approval for clinical trials of 3BP on hepatocellular carcinoma and other cancers. But the wheels of FDA approval turn very slowly.

These discoveries have sparked a wave of therapies aiming at metabolism rather than genetics alone. Approaches like ketogenic diets, which lower glucose in the blood and raise ketones (an alternative energy source for healthy cells), are now studied in clinics worldwide. Researchers are testing drugs and compounds that disrupt the abnormal fuel flow inside cancer cells or restore healthier mitochondrial function. Some clinics offer 3BP infusions or combine metabolic strategies with standard treatments to amplify results and reduce side effects.

Of course, these ideas stir up debate. Most oncologists still follow treatment guidelines focused on genetics and rapidly dividing cells. Insurance rarely covers metabolic therapies outside clinical trials. Many doctors worry about safety or lack of long-term results for these newer tools. The "standard of care" is slow to change because it relies on large, multi-year studies before approving new protocols. Patients get caught in the middle—wanting to try metabolism-based approaches but told by their care teams that there isn't enough evidence yet or that it's not "approved." For many, though,

Warburg's legacy and Dr. Ko's work open new windows of hope where doors once seemed locked shut.

The Rise of Repurposed Drugs: From Dewormers to Oncology

If someone had told me several years ago that a dog dewormer would become a beacon of hope for people with cancer, I would have laughed or thought it was a wild rumor. Yet, here we are—fenbendazole, originally designed to rid pets of parasites, is now at the heart of countless cancer discussions. It started quietly, with whispers in online support groups.

Then came the story of Joe Tippens. He was diagnosed with small cell lung cancer and told he had three months to live. Out of options, Joe began taking fenbendazole, alongside his current treatment and vitamins and supplements. His scans eventually showed no evidence of disease (NED)[2]. (His case remains anecdotal and cannot officially establish causation.) Joe's story went viral, and suddenly, desperate patients everywhere wanted to understand what, exactly, was going on. Forums filled with posts about dosing schedules, brands, and lab results shared by real people, not just scientists in white coats.

Ivermectin followed a similar path. Once recognized mostly as a treatment for river blindness or scabies, it's now discussed in podcasts, patient groups, and even published cancer research. I've seen caregivers in online forums compare notes about using ivermectin as an adjunct to chemotherapy, sometimes in combination with fenbendazole. These conversations rarely start with "miracle cure" claims. Instead, they begin with questions: "Has anyone tried this alongside immunotherapy?" "What side effects should I watch for?" "How do I avoid fake products?" The sharing is raw, practical, and driven by hope—but also by caution.

This shift isn't just about desperation. There's real scientific logic behind repurposing drugs. Many medications created for one purpose have hidden properties that only show up when tested in new ways. Fenbendazole interferes with microtubules—tiny structures that help cells divide—similar to some chemotherapy drugs, but with a different toxicity profile. Ivermectin impacts cellular signaling and may disrupt cancer cell metabolism or even trigger cell death under certain conditions[3]. These effects are now being studied more seriously by scientists. Researchers look for drugs with proven safety records in animals or humans, low cost, and the ability to hit cancer cells through unique biological pathways.

However, this rapid rise of repurposed drugs comes with regulatory hurdles and safety concerns. Unlike new cancer drugs, veterinary medications like fenbendazole aren't approved for use in humans by the FDA or similar agencies elsewhere. That means no pharmaceutical company stands behind their use for cancer, and nobody is monitoring for side effects in a clinical way. Patients often have to source veterinary medications themselves, raising questions about purity, authenticity, and dosage. Regulatory bodies issue warnings about buying medicine online or using animal products outside their intended purpose. The safety net is thin, and people must weigh risks against potential benefits. If you should decide to use a product formulated for animals, I suggest a thorough look at the anecdotal reports and product reviews.

The evidence for these protocols stretches across a spectrum—from powerful personal stories and early lab studies to ongoing clinical trials and published case reports. Anecdotes like Joe Tippens' draw attention. They spark curiosity and sometimes even push researchers to study old drugs in new ways. However, there's a big leap between a single story and scientific proof. Some patients experience side effects or no benefit at all, while others see remarkable results. Rigorous research takes time and money—something many off-patent drugs don't attract easily. Even so, the explosion of interest keeps fueling studies, some of which are now appearing in respected medical journals.

In this space between hope and hard science, people like you are left making tough decisions—balancing peer advice with research, regulatory warnings with stories of survival, and always searching for that next piece of information that could tip the scales.

How Patient Forums Shape Protocol Adoption

When you step into a cancer patient forum for the first time, the energy is electric—raw questions, real worries, and a sense of urgency that you simply won't find in sterile medical offices. These online communities—whether on Facebook, Reddit, or patient-specific message boards—become lifelines. People swap details about what they're trying, what works, and what to avoid. You might see someone post their daily supplement list, complete with dosing and timing, or share a photo of their medication bottle for others to cross-check. The conversations often move at breakneck speed, with new protocols emerging from the collective efforts of patients eager to help one another. What's especially striking is how quickly an idea or regimen can spread. One person shares a result, and within days, dozens are tweaking their own routines, comparing notes, and reporting back. There's a kind of grassroots clinical trial happening every hour—imperfect, but undeniably powerful.

Peer support in these spaces is more than emotional; it's practical. When conventional care leaves gaps, patients fill them for each other. Dosing charts circulate—sometimes created in a spreadsheet, sometimes scrawled on notebook paper and scanned for the group. You see color-coded tables matching weights with fenbendazole doses, or ivermectin schedules adapted from veterinary recommendations but converted for human use. Someone will always step in to double-check calculations, warn about possible interactions, or point out a missed detail. It feels almost like a team effort, with everyone invested in each other's outcomes. When someone posts about a side effect or setback, responses pour in—tips, gentle warnings, or simple words of encouragement. For many, this support becomes as important as any pill or protocol.

Still, the value of anecdotal evidence has its limits. Individual stories—while often inspiring—can create false hope or confusion. One person's "miracle" can become another person's disappointment, especially if details get lost or exaggerated along the way. You'll see disagreements pop up: Was the improvement really from fenbendazole, or did it coincide with a new chemo round? Did someone's cancer shrink because of a protocol, or was it a fluke? These forums don't provide controlled trials; they provide snapshots, sometimes fuzzy, sometimes clear. Sorting through the noise can be exhausting, but for many, it's better than silence.

The anecdotal evidence is overwhelming and impossible to ignore. That's why documented, credible case studies are so vital. When someone posts before-and-after scan results, or shares lab data with dates and doctor notes attached, the conversation shifts. People pay closer attention to details: cancer type, stage, concurrent treatments, timeframes. You see members encourage others to keep logs or journals, not just for themselves but to help the group build a clearer picture of what works—and what doesn't. These documented stories carry more weight, not just in the forum but sometimes even in clinical research. Researchers have begun using patient reports as starting points for formal studies. Every chart, diary, or scan shared adds to a growing body of real-world evidence.

Community wisdom, at its best, speeds up the feedback loop between discovery and outcome. Protocols get refined in real time; mistakes are caught and corrected faster than isolated trial and error. Sometimes what starts as a hunch or rumor gets shaped into a protocol that researchers eventually notice. Other times, the group's collective skepticism helps weed out unsafe or ineffective ideas. The power of these communities lies not just in numbers, but in their ability to crowdsource solutions that might otherwise be overlooked, and to demand better answers—together.

Distinguishing Science from Hype: A Guide to Evaluating Claims

Sorting through cancer information is like walking through a minefield—everywhere you turn, there's a new miracle cure or cautionary tale. Some days, it feels impossible to separate hope from hype, especially when you're tired and craving answers. It's easy to get swept up in stories, especially when you want so much for them to be true. But real healing requires more than wishful thinking; it demands a clear eye and a steady hand.

I've learned to slow down and ask hard questions before believing any claim. The first tool I use is simple skepticism—not cynicism, but the willingness to pause and ask, "Who's saying this? What's their background? Do they stand to profit?" Concrete science rarely hides behind paywalls or aggressive marketing. If a website pushes products before providing evidence, or if every sentence ends with "Buy now!"—that's a flashing warning light. Credible sources cite research, not just stories. When you see references to journals, university studies, or clinical trials, check if they link to the actual studies or just mention them vaguely. Good science encourages scrutiny and welcomes questions.

Whenever I encounter a new protocol, I run it through a mental checklist. Does the person making the claim have medical or scientific training? Are actual patient outcomes documented, or is the evidence only anecdotal? Is there a plausible mechanism for why this protocol should work, based on what we know about cancer biology? Are side effects and risks discussed openly? If someone claims a treatment is totally safe for everyone, that's another red flag—no real therapy is risk-free. Avoid sources that promise 100% success or insist doctors are hiding "the cure." Real medicine is nuanced and admits uncertainty.

Misinformation often carries certain patterns. Scams flourish where desperation lives. Beware of anyone who insists you must act quickly or risk missing out. If a product is only available through one website or "exclusive" provider, skepticism is warranted. Watch for testimonials with dramatic before-and-after photos but no verifiable medical records. If negative experiences or questions are deleted from forums, something isn't right. Reputable communities allow open debate and are transparent about both successes and failures.

There is a fine line between balanced hope and dangerous optimism. It's healthy to seek possibilities, but not to the point of abandoning reason or ignoring real risks. Hope should be informed, not blind. The best advocates for alternative therapies are those who acknowledge what isn't yet known, who share both promising results and honest setbacks. Surround yourself with people—online or in person—who value truth over hype.

If you want to sharpen your discernment, there are resources that can help. Look for organizations that specialize in evaluating alternative cancer therapies with a critical eye. Some cancer non-profits publish guides on questions to ask about new treatments. Medical librarians at major hospitals can help you find real research articles. Stay connected to support groups (see Resources) where skepticism is encouraged, not punished. Keep your trusted healthcare providers in the loop about anything you're considering—they can provide context and may help spot risks you might miss.

Navigating this landscape takes courage and care. The good news is that with the right mindset and tools, you can protect yourself from false promises while staying open to breakthroughs grounded in genuine evidence. This balance—staying hopeful but never naive—will serve you and your loved ones well as you continue forward with strength and clarity.

Chapter 2
Metabolic Therapies — Diet and Beyond

The Glucose-Ketone Index: Dr. Thomas Seyfried's Cancer Starvation Model

One thing that truly shook me out of my old way of thinking was learning that you can actually measure whether your body is fueling cancer—or starving it. Imagine you could track not just your blood sugar, but the balance between sugar and ketones, and use this information to shift your internal environment away from what supports tumor growth. This isn't just a theory; it's a tool you can use at home. Dr. Thomas Seyfried, a respected Boston College researcher in the metabolic approach to cancer, developed what's called the Glucose-Ketone Index (GKI). For a lot of people, this number becomes a lifeline—something solid to hold onto when everything else feels uncertain.

Let's break down what the GKI really is. Your body can run on two main fuels: glucose (sugar) and ketones (produced from fat when glucose is scarce). Cancer cells thrive on glucose—they can't survive on ketones. Dr. Seyfried's research suggests that if you lower your glucose enough, while raising ketones, you might slow cancer growth or even shrink tumors. The GKI is a simple ratio that compares your blood glucose level to your blood ketone level. To calculate it, you measure both using fingerstick monitors, one that measures glucose (the same kind people with diabetes use), and another for measuring ketones. Then you divide your glucose measurement by your ketone measurement.

The calculation method differs slightly, depending on which measurement system your country uses:

In the USA, glucose is measured in mg/dL (milligrams per deciliter), while ketones are typically measured in mmol/L (millimoles per liter). To calculate your GKI, you need to convert your glucose reading to mmol/L by dividing it by 18, then divide that number by your ketone reading. Example: If your glucose is 80 mg/dL (which equals 4.4 mmol/L) and your beta-hydroxybutyrate (your main blood ketone) is 2.0 mmol/L, your GKI is 4.4 ÷ 2.0 = 2.2.

In the UK and Canada, among others, both glucose and ketones are measured in mmol/L (millimoles per liter). To calculate your GKI, you simply divide your glucose reading by your ketone reading. Example: If your glucose is 4.4 mmol/L and your ketones are 2.0 mmol/L, your GKI is 4.4 ÷ 2.0 = 2.2.

The lower your GKI number, the more you are in a metabolic state that may have therapeutic benefits. Dr. Thomas Seyfried's clinical work suggests a GKI goal of around 1.0–2.0 for those with active cancer, though individual needs can vary.

Why does this matter? Well, tumors don't just "like" sugar—they depend on it. By keeping your GKI low, you create a metabolic environment where cancer cells struggle but healthy cells—able to use ketones—can keep going strong. This approach is different from traditional calorie restriction or simply "eating less sugar." It's about changing the ratio so that glucose is low and ketones are elevated at the same time, not just one or the other.

Monitoring your GKI at home isn't as technical or scary as it sounds. You don't need a lab coat or an advanced degree—just curiosity and a bit of patience. You'll need two tools: a blood glucose meter and a ketone meter (some devices test both from the same drop of blood). Both are available online or at most pharmacies. The "Keto Mojo" is one meter that measures both glucose and ketones. For accuracy, always use blood measurements, not urine strips, as those are less reliable for tracking real-time ketone levels.

The third thing you'll need is most likely a dietary change to produce ketones in your body. This happens naturally with very low carbohydrate intake. Later in this chapter, we'll cover the specifics of diet, and the simple way you can achieve ketone production.

Here's how to measure your GKI: each morning before eating, wash your hands well (residues can throw off results), prick your finger with the lancet, and collect a drop of blood on each test strip—one for glucose, one for ketones. Write down the numbers or use a tracking app. Convert glucose readings from mg/dL to mmol/L if needed (divide by 18). Then divide the glucose number by the ketone number to get your GKI. If you check at the same time daily (in a fasted state), you get a clear picture of how your dietary changes are working.

Some studies, including lab and small clinical trials, show that maintaining a low GKI might slow tumor progression, make chemo or radiation work better, or even help some people reach remission[4]. Dr. Seyfried's work is widely cited in metabolic cancer circles for showing how ketogenic diets can lower GKI and impact tumor metabolism. However, there's debate in the oncology world about how much this translates to everyone with cancer. Critics say that not all cancers respond the same way; some may adapt to burn other fuels besides glucose, like fatty acids, although Dr. Seyfried has said that he hasn't found a cancer yet that can survive in the absence of glucose *and* glutamine. Others worry about weight loss in already frail patients or possible ketoacidosis (though this is rare in non-diabetics); **this**

is why a nutrient-dense way of eating is necessary. Still, many oncologists acknowledge that keeping blood sugar stable and avoiding spikes is almost always helpful, especially for those dealing with 'insulin resistance' or on steroids during treatment.

It would be fair to note that while Dr. Seyfried's metabolic theory does have supporting research, large-scale randomized controlled trials in humans are still limited, and will most likely remain so (since there is no potential mega-money drug involved); most evidence comes from animal studies, case reports, and small clinical trials.

For further understanding of this, here's an excerpt of a conversation between Dr. Seyfried and Jim Puplava of FinancialSense.com:

> ***Jim Puplava:***
>
> *Why do you think the medical profession has been reluctant to even look at this? You would think if there was a new protocol for curing somebody, whether it's proton beam radiation or something like that, the medical profession would embrace it. But they seem reluctant. Why is that?*
>
> ***Dr. Thomas Seyfried:***
>
> *They can't make money on it. It's not complicated. I want you to remember one thing, and remember it's important: revenue generation first, patient outcome second. That's it. You have a multi-billion-dollar industry making massive amounts of money using poisonous chemicals, radiation, surgical mutilation, and all this kind of stuff. Then you come along with something that can get the job done without toxicity, but you can't make any money on it. How excited are you going to be about that?*

The entire interview[5] mentioned above is well worth reading.

The mainstream oncology community generally views ketogenic diets as an adjunct or experimental approach rather than a standalone treatment. But, if someone were fighting cancer, my view is it certainly can't hurt, there's evidence that a keto diet will increase the effectiveness of conventional treatments, and that person will almost certainly get healthier in the meantime.

When setting GKI goals for yourself as someone with cancer, context matters. Dr. Seyfried suggests aiming for a GKI below 2.0 for aggressive therapeutic intent, especially during active treatment phases. Some patients report benefits even with GKIs in the 2–3 range if they can't tolerate stricter diets. For prevention or maintenance after remission, keeping it under 5 might be enough for some people. What matters most is consistency—small daily choices add up over time.

Reflection Exercise: Tracking Your Own Numbers

Get yourself a notebook or open a new note on your phone labeled "My GKI Log." For two weeks, record your morning fasting glucose and ketones each day. Note any changes you make in your eating habits—more healthy fats, fewer carbs—and watch how your numbers shift. How does your body respond when you skip dessert? Does stress affect your readings? Write down not just the numbers but how you feel physically and emotionally each day. After two weeks, look for trends: Are you moving toward a lower GKI? Do you feel more energetic or clearer-headed? If so, celebrate those wins—they're proof that small changes can make a real difference.

Navigating cancer is about reclaiming whatever control you can over your body and health. The Glucose-Ketone Index gives you a window into your metabolism that anyone can use at home without waiting for permission from experts or insurance companies. It's one way to turn fear into action and confusion into something measurable—something that puts power back in your hands, even if just a little bit at a time.

Implementing a Therapeutic Ketogenic Diet: Practical Steps and Pitfalls

When one first encounters the ketogenic diet, it can seem daunting, with new terms like "macros," "keto flu," and fat bombs. Transitioning from decades of eating bagels, breakfast cereals, potatoes and pasta to a high-fat, low-carb diet can feel alien, but this shift doesn't have to happen overnight. In fact, making the transition gradually over four to six weeks can result in fewer unpleasantries like the keto flu, and it gives your microbiome a chance to adjust. Gut bugs that have been eating lots of junk food don't belong there; gut bugs that thrive on meat and fatty acids do. If you rush the transition, you'll likely face significant physical and emotional hurdles. So, take your time.

Below is a suggested timeline. As you work your way through it, eat meat and the fat that comes with it, especially beef, bacon, eggs, and/or fish at every meal.

WEEK	FOODS TO ELIMINATE
Week 1	Eliminate obvious junk foods (cakes, cookies, candies, etc.).
Week 2	Eliminate grains, such as breads, pasta, and hot and cold cereals. These are high in carbohydrates and anti-nutrients. Also eliminate seed oils; they are inflammatory.
Week 3	Eliminate high-carbohydrate vegetables such as white and sweet potatoes.
Week 4	Eliminate high-carbohydrate fruits, such as bananas and pineapple.
Note	You can stretch weeks two, three and four out an additional week if you like, to round out your transition to six or seven weeks.

Start by eliminating obvious sugars—ditch desserts, sodas, and juices. Replace carb-heavy breakfasts with eggs or Greek yogurt. Each week, drop off more carbs and replace with options like cauliflower in place of rice or extra green veggies instead of potatoes. Add healthy fats: beef tallow, bacon grease, lard, oils like coconut, olive, avocado, or walnut. Watch out for hidden sugars and seed oils (like canola, soy, and corn) in sauces and dressings.

Your body needs time to adjust. Fatigue or irritability during the first weeks is normal—it's your metabolism transitioning from burning sugar to fat, and your body is recovering from carb addiction. Don't stress if you notice an energy dip or increased cravings. Staying well-hydrated; adding a bit of salt or a clean electrolyte powder or drops to your water helps because low-carb diets flush out water that your body has been retaining, and with it go your electrolytes like sodium, potassium, and magnesium. Bone broth can be especially helpful during this adjustment. If you are taking medication you will want your doctor to monitor those levels so you don't end up over-medicated as your body works more efficiently eating low-carb.

Macro ratios sound complex, but quickly become second nature. For cancer therapy, aim for about 70-80% calories from fat, 15-20% from protein, and 5-10% from carbs. You don't have to eat plain butter (but that's okay too). Include fatty meats (especially beef), oily fish like salmon, mackerel, sardines, and herring, and eggs. For carbs, stick to low carb versions, like leafy greens, broccoli, zucchini, and non-starchy veggies. Keep protein moderate and fat high—too much protein can push you out of ketosis since excess converts to glucose. Use a food tracking app or journal initially to help visualize your intake and avoid accidental carb creep.

Meal planning is essential. Without ready keto-friendly options, it's easy to fall back on old habits in moments of hunger. Batch cook proteins like chicken thighs or chili with ground beef and cauliflower rice. Stock up on hard-boiled eggs, cheese sticks, and roasted nuts for quick snacks. Salads with olive oil-based dressings and grilled chicken are filling and fast. If cooking isn't your thing, many keto meal delivery services and simple online recipes exist.

Several common mistakes can derail your progress. One is "dirty keto," focusing solely on macronutrient targets but eating mostly processed meats, artificial sweeteners, and chemical-laden snacks. You might stay in ketosis, but your body needs real nutrients, especially during therapy. **Prioritize whole foods or minimally processed foods**. Another common error is ignoring electrolytes. As mentioned previously, eating low carb makes your kidneys release more sodium and water; inadequate electrolyte replacement can cause dizziness, weakness, or cramps. Daily broth or a commercial electrolyte supplement can prevent this.

What is a whole food? A natural unprocessed, or minimally-processed food, usually with one ingredient. <u>Examples</u>: Beef contains: beef. Cauliflower contains: cauliflower.

What is a minimally processed food? A whole food that has been slightly and gently altered (such as by washing, freezing, or pasteurizing) for convenience or extended shelf life. These foods generally retain all or almost all of their natural nutrition. Examples: produce that has been washed, cut, chopped, and/or frozen. Eggs that have been washed and/or pasteurized. Pasteurized dairy products.

The social side of eating low-carb may be the toughest challenge. Friends and family often offer carb-heavy comfort foods, and declining can feel awkward. Explain your dietary choices and goals; most people will be supportive if they understand why it matters. If not, quietly stick to your plan and contribute keto-friendly dishes to social gatherings when possible.

Keto-adaptation symptoms like headaches, nausea, fatigue, and the infamous "keto flu" are common but temporary, usually lasting a few days to a couple of weeks. Symptoms improve as your body switches to fat burning. Increase water and salt intake. If constipation arises, magnesium citrate or a bit more olive oil can help during the transition. For sleep disruptions or anxiety, make sure you're eating enough fat and not overdoing caffeine, especially later in the day.

If you're using keto therapeutically—especially for cancer—lab monitoring is crucial. Before making big dietary changes, get baseline labs: fasting blood sugar, insulin, liver and kidney function, inflammatory markers like CRP and/or Sed Rate, and for whatever medications you may be taking. Recheck important labs after a few weeks to track your body's response. If you monitor your weight, note that rapid early loss is mostly water, not fat or muscle. In fact, a ketogenic diet can help to protect against the loss of muscle and bone (unlike a standard American diet), and fat loss typically follows the water loss over time.

Professional support can be invaluable. Even if your oncologist isn't familiar with the ketogenic diet for cancer, a ketogenic dietitian or ketogenic nutritionist can customize a safe, effective plan for you and monitor potential issues. (Regular dieticians or nutritionists are typically not trained to support ketogenic diets.) Some cancer centers offer integrative oncology services with nutrition counseling; ask your provider or search for remote specialists if needed. If your doctor, dietician, or nutritionist tells you that you need lots of carbohydrates, take this book in, and let them read the Therapeutic Ketogenic Diet and Carnivore sections of this chapter.

If your doctor refuses to educate himself or herself, find another one. If you can't find another one, due to insurance limitations or other constraints, implement a low-carb way of eating anyway. I don't say that flippantly or lightly, as working with your medical team is always best; however, there is no adequate substitute for basic human nutrition—it's that important—and it is simply not taught in medical schools (that's a whole other discussion). **And, for goodness' sakes, do not eat the high-carb sugary goodies and juices offered by many cancer treatment centers (insert eye-roll and hand to forehead).**

Eating this way may feel unusual at first, but, over time, routines develop and it gets easier. You may notice steadier energy, sharper thinking, and perhaps even improvements in your lab results or appetite control. Remember, perfection is not the goal, but being patience and consistency as you build new habits, one meal at a time.

Carnivore Diet for Cancer: When, Why, and How

You've likely heard about the carnivore diet—maybe from a podcast, a Facebook group, or a daring friend who eats only animal foods. I was skeptical about it because, like just about every other person on earth, I was told we need to eat a variety of plants to get all of our nutrition. But after I looked into it more closely, I discovered that not only do we not need to eat plants, but eating plants can be contrary to health goals, since they all contain antinutrients, some more than others. The carnivore diet, especially in the context of cancer therapy, is simple: you eat only animal foods—meat, fish, eggs, and sometimes dairy if tolerated. There are no grains, beans, fruit, or even minimal salad. This low-carb approach cuts nearly all carbohydrates and plant-based anti-nutrients, focusing instead on protein and fat. While it's about restricting glucose (fuel for tumors), it's also about simplicity and eliminating foods that might trigger irritation or inflammation. It dramatically simplifies things, so if you're overwhelmed, or you want to ensure that you are producing ketones, you might want to consider eating carnivore.

Nutritional completeness is a common concern. Many fear you'll lack vitamins, minerals, or fiber—but the need for fiber is a myth and is overblown. Once plants are removed and fat intake increases, digestion adapts. A carnivore diet is **nutritionally complete**. Many carnivore eaters report improved, regular bowel movements, and less gas and bloating. Eating "nose-to-tail" (including organ meats and bone broths alongside muscle meat) provides a wide spectrum of bioavailable nutrients. Beef liver is a powerhouse of vitamin A, B vitamins, iron, zinc, and more, while eggs and seafood provide choline, selenium, and omega-3s. A variety of animal foods covers micronutrient requirements; most carnivores just supplement with a bit of extra salt or electrolytes, and sometimes magnesium. Organ meat is optional, but it is very nutrient-dense, and perfect for days you may not feel like eating due to your treatment regimen.

Carnivore eating offers benefits beyond simplicity. For those with cancer, the main arguments are inflammation reduction, eliminating a major tumor fuel source, keeping the digestive tract calm, and reducing inflammation. Plants contain lectins, oxalates, phytates, and other anti-nutrients, which may irritate the gut or reduce absorption of key minerals. Many people notice less joint pain, better mental clarity, and fewer digestive symptoms after removing these compounds. While clinical trials are limited (again, there's no monetary incentive for these studies), case reports and cautious physician use are increasing, especially with patients who struggle on ketogenic diets. Carnivore can be simpler to follow with no counting carbs, macros, or food tracking: just eat meat and fat when hungry, and eat until you're full. As a result, ketones rise, blood sugar and insulin stay low, and many experience more energy and improved mood.

Transitioning fully to carnivore requires some preparation. Following the same transition schedule we discussed earlier, you gradually reduce plant foods, replacing them with more fatty meat, fatty fish, and eggs, and using broth for electrolytes can help. Carb cravings and missing crunchy foods can last a week or two, but usually subside. As with keto, hydration and salt are essential—without plants, your body isn't dealing with anti-nutrients, and retaining water, so you excrete more sodium. Add salt to meals, sip broth, and opt for fattier cuts of meat like ribeye, pork belly, or salmon rather than just lean meats, which can leave you fatigued. Optionally, include organs like liver or heart weekly, and make broth from bones. Though unusual to some, these foods were dietary staples for our ancient human ancestors[6] and traditional cultures, and offer nutrients you won't find in smoothies. Bone broth supplies collagen and minerals, aiding gut and tissue repair—especially useful for those recovering from cancer treatments. Full-fat dairy can be added if tolerated.

Who benefits from carnivore?

Those with severe food sensitivities, autoimmune problems, or gut issues often improve quickly. For cancer patients struggling with digestive symptoms, animal foods can be more tolerable and are nutrient-dense. Lower inflammation, improved energy, and easier weight management are common. Concerns about kidney health are generally overstated; unless advanced kidney disease is present, high protein intake isn't shown to cause harm—and even then, proper hydration and mineral balance can help. Cholesterol worries also tend to fade, as triglycerides tend to drop and HDL rises; most see heart health indicators improve after the adjustment period.

Cancer and Carnivore

The internet is bubbling with people whose cancer went into remission by eating a carnivore diet, with or without standard treatments. Following are just two of those. You can hear them tell their story, in their own words, on YouTube. There's a QR code to scan, or a link to visit.

Jason improved esophageal cancer, which had metastasized throughout his body, after being told he had just 3-12 months to live. Telling his story 15 months after diagnosis, he has renewed hope.

https://youtu.be/ciClMZsfhqQ?si=7zu_3OACoF75MboO

David put his incurable, non-operable very-high-stage-4 blood cancer into remission, and is healing the damage caused by previous chemotherapies, with the carnivore diet.

SCAN ME

https://youtu.be/-LK2yyPwgqU?si=lqRTVDIcIY-IbfTi

A few misconceptions to clarify: You don't need to eat only steak—ground meat, poultry, fish, and eggs all fit the diet. There's no need to force-feed or calorie restrict; eat to satiety. If you're hesitant about dropping fruits or vegetables entirely, after your initial four to six week transition, try a 30-day experiment of just carnivore and judge how you feel—you can always reintroduce foods later. If fiber is a concern, remember: your gut bacteria will adapt, thriving on protein and fats instead of plants, just like our ancient human ancestors. Issues like constipation or diarrhea frequently resolve, not worsen, for those who stick with carnivore.

In closing, metabolic therapies offer practical, hands-on ways to positively influence your body's internal environment—tipping the odds in your favor. Whether you choose keto, carnivore, or something in between, the most important factor is to listen to your body (beyond any transition cravings) and make informed, deliberate choices. The next chapter delves farther into the metabolic realm with advanced metabolic therapies.

Chapter 3
Advanced Metabolic and Adjunctive Therapies

Press-Pulse Therapy: Theory and Application

Imagine watching a campfire burn down: a difference exists between a slow flame and a sudden flare. That image helps explain the press-pulse approach in cancer therapy. Rather than overwhelming your body with drastic or constant change, the strategy uses steady, ongoing pressure to starve cancer cells ("press"), paired with strategic, short-term, high-impact bursts ("pulse") that hit tumor vulnerabilities—all with minimal stress for healthy tissue.

The "press-pulse" model, borrowed from ecology, balances persistent and intermittent interventions to wipe out unwanted populations. For cancer, "press" means ongoing metabolic stress—most often a sustained ketogenic diet (with or without calorie restriction) that lowers blood sugar and elevates ketones. Cancer cells, heavily reliant on glucose and unable to efficiently use ketones for fuel, struggle in this environment, while healthy cells adapt and thrive. The goal isn't starvation, but shifting your metabolism until your body becomes a hostile environment for cancer.

The "pulse" involves targeted, intermittent stress layered on the foundation of ongoing metabolic therapy. Pulses might be 24–48 hour fasts—denying cancer cells nutrients and triggering **autophagy** (cellular cleanup). They could be pulsed high-dose vitamin C, or hyperbaric oxygen therapy (HBOT). (You'll hear Dr. Thomas Seyfried speak of 6-Diazo-5-oxo-L-norleucine (DON), a glutamine blocker, or glutaminase inhibitors, which in the USA are used only in research and clinical trials and not available to the general public.)

Pulses are usually timed for maximum impact—sometimes alongside chemotherapy schedules, or if blood tests indicate tumor progression. Properly applied pulses jolt tumor metabolism, but are short enough to avoid overtaxing you.

In practice, a "press" might be the ketogenic diet you follow daily, with regularly lower blood sugar and elevated ketones. Every week or couple of weeks, you might add longer fasting, or HBOT. The intention is always to target the cancer—not to push your body to exhaustion.

Home-based press-pulse therapy is achievable with basic self-monitoring. Start by learning to check blood glucose and ketone levels with a fingerstick monitor and record the results. Keep glucose low (often under 90 mg/dL) and ketones moderate to high (1.0–3.0 mmol/L)—the backbone of your "press." If you're new to fasting, start gradually with overnight fasts (12 hours) before building to longer stretches if tolerated, always watching how you feel.

Do your homework and consult with a knowledgeable healthcare provider if possible. Some interventions—such as supplements or medications—may be available over the counter, while others require participation in clinical trials. Dosing and timing are key: for instance, high-dose vitamin C might be paired with chemotherapy sessions (check for drug interactions and contraindications). Monitor for side effects like fatigue or digestive changes, and adjust your regimen as needed.

The "pulse" portion of press pulse therapy is the strategic and timely (not constant, which could be harmful), repression of glutamine. Some integrative and metabolic oncology discussions include fenbendazole and mebendazole as metabolic modifiers that may be useful in a press–pulse style approach, but this is **not the same as documented glutamine pulsing protocols** used in formal research. A review article[7] notes that maximal benefit of 6-Diazo-5-oxo-L-norleucine (DON) and mebendazole occurred when used alongside a ketogenic diet in certain experimental settings, not as standalone or well-defined pulses. DON is not approved or available in the United States for cancer treatment (see Important Online Resource for Press Pulse Therapy, below). Dr. Seyfried has stated (at 0:11:07 in the transcript) that his research team has successfully tested mebendazole, not fenbendazole, as a pulse for glutamine[8].

Clinical and anecdotal evidence on press-pulse is promising but still evolving. Some studies and patient reports note tumor shrinkage or stabilization when combining strict dietary oversight with intermittent fasting or metabolic-targeted supplements, with additional benefits like improved energy or sleep during the "press" phase alone. Not all patients respond the same—cancer is highly individualized—but accumulating evidence supports the use of press-pulse techniques to slow progression and enhance outcomes, often with fewer side effects.

If you are fortunate enough you might even find an integrative physician or oncologist to help you implement press pulse therapy. Point them in the direction of Dr. Thomas Seyfried's press pulse therapy; I believe he is willing to share exact his protocol with physicians.

Important Online Resource for Press Pulse Therapy

However, even if you are unable to locate an integrative physician to help you implement press pulse therapy, the KetoForCancer Skool community purports to help people to implement the press pulse therapy, and includes diet guidance. It was created by Johnny Rockermeier, sidekick to Dr. Thomas Seyfried, and is reasonably priced at $65/year; there is also a monthly subscription option (as of this writing)—and they offer a 1-week FREE trial (I am not affiliated in any way). It also purports to **show you how to get DON legally in your country**. For more info, visit https://skool.com/ketoforcancer

Interactive Exercise: Press-Pulse Journal

Keep a journal of symptoms: note energy levels, pain scores, sleep quality, appetite changes, new side effects, mood shifts—these can sometimes reveal subtle improvements or problems before labs do. Write down how you feel, physically and emotionally. Every two weeks, review the log: What helps or hinders your well-being? Are tumor markers or lab values improving? Share this log at check-ins with your provider or a trusted caregiver.

If you encounter lower energy, rapid weight loss, or ongoing fatigue, ease up on the protocol or space out the pulses further. Personalized adjustments aren't failures—they're vital to a therapy that must be tailored to your body's response.

Over time, you'll find which combinations and timing work best for you. Some thrive with shorter, more frequent pulses; others do well remaining longer in ketosis with less frequent additions.

Press-pulse therapy is flexible, grounded in cancer metabolism science, and puts powerful tools in your hands for managing your internal environment. By combining steady metabolic stress with periodic targeted interventions, and tracking your responses, you can systematically support your body's resilience and make conditions ever less favorable for cancer cells.

3-Bromopyruvate (3BP): Young Hee Ko's Innovation

The first time I heard about 3-bromopyruvate (3BP), it sounded almost too simple. Here was a small molecule, discovered and refined by Dr. Young

Hee Ko, that seemed to strike at the very heart of what makes cancer so stubborn. If you're new to 3BP, picture it as a metabolic disruptor—a "wrench in the gears" for cancer's unique way of fueling itself. Instead of trying to blast cancer with toxins or cut it out completely, 3BP sneaks in and sabotages the cell's ability to use sugar for energy. Cancer cells love sugar. They thrive on it, gobbling up glucose and spitting out lactic acid at rates that normal cells simply don't. This is known as the Warburg Effect, an odd metabolic trick that lets tumors grow faster and survive in places where oxygen is low. What makes 3BP so clever is how it finds its way into cancer cells using the very transporters those cells have upregulated to bring in more fuel. Once inside, it blocks the machinery that turns sugar into usable energy and stops lactic acid from being pumped out, leading to an acidic, toxic mess that only the cancer cell can't handle. Your healthy cells—using fewer of these transporters—mostly get left alone.

It's one thing to have a theory; it's another to see it in action. In lab studies, 3BP has consistently outperformed traditional chemotherapies. Scientists have tested it on more than a hundred cancer cell lines—liver, colon, breast, brain, and others—and found that 3BP shuts down energy production so effectively that cancer cells die off, sometimes even when chemo couldn't touch them. Animal studies show similar promise. Mice with aggressive tumors treated with 3BP experienced shrinkage or complete disappearance of their tumors, often without the toxic fallout that chemo brings. But animal studies only go so far. The leap to humans is always tricky, and the data is still building. Early clinical cases, especially those treated at specialized centers like Dayspring Cancer Clinic in Scottsdale Arizona, show real-world promise. Some patients who had run out of options—chemo failed, radiation did nothing, immunotherapy didn't work—saw their tumors shrink or stabilize after starting 3BP therapy, often alongside a ketogenic diet to starve the cancer further.

The First Human Application of 3BP

Yvar Verhoeven's Story

Yvar Verhoeven[9] was a 16-year-old from the Netherlands diagnosed with fibrolamellar hepatocellular carcinoma, a rare form of liver cancer for which there is no known treatment other than transplantation. He did not qualify for transplantation and was initially treated with sorafenib, the standard liver cancer drug, but any benefits were short-lived.

Treatment with 3BP began in February 2009, administered by Dr. Young Hee Ko in collaboration with radiologist Thomas Vogl at the University Hospital Frankfurt in Germany.

The treatment showed remarkable initial results. Yvar's very poor appetite was quickly reversed, his enlarged spleen was drastically reduced, indications of tumor death were evident, and regeneration of liver tissue was observed. By summer he had begun to regain his physical strength.

A photograph was taken on Yvar's 18th birthday, September 9, 2009, at his home in the Netherlands after his 7th treatment with 3BP. This was particularly meaningful as he had been told he would never make it to his 17th birthday. He recovered sufficiently to tour the United States and make a presentation with Dr. Ko.

However, despite regeneration of liver cells, his liver functions were overloaded and couldn't cope with the rapid destruction of tumor cells. The liver couldn't detoxify dead cancer cell debris fast enough. Though the cancer had been eradicated, and he lived much longer than expected with an improved quality of life, Yvar died two years after his initial diagnosis.

Getting access to 3BP isn't as simple as picking up a prescription at the pharmacy. It's not FDA-approved for general use in the United States or most other countries. Instead, clinics that operate under Institutional Review Board (IRB) oversight for investigational therapies may use it. This means you can't just ask your local oncologist for 3BP; you need to seek out specialized centers, often traveling and paying out of pocket. Legal status varies by country and even by state. Some patients outside the U.S. have flown to Europe or Asia for compassionate-use programs. The investigational status means that, while there's growing evidence for efficacy and safety, there are no guarantees of insurance coverage or easy access. If you're considering 3BP, start by contacting clinics with IRB-approved protocols and ask about patient eligibility, pre-treatment evaluations, and estimated costs. Dayspring Cancer Center in Scottsdale Arizona is one such clinic. Dr. Dickens there worked directly with Dr. Ko for five years.

Safety always comes first. While 3BP seems less toxic than many chemotherapy drugs, it's still a potent metabolic inhibitor and must be administered by experienced professionals. The intravenous route is standard, requiring careful dosing and slow infusions to avoid irritation or complications. Common side effects include mild fever, chills, fatigue, or gastrointestinal upset—usually manageable with supportive care. Serious adverse events are rare but possible; inappropriately high doses or improper administration can cause tissue irritation or kidney stress. This isn't a therapy to try at home or with unregulated sources. If you have liver or kidney problems, make sure your care team monitors your labs closely before and during treatment.

Combining 3BP with other therapies is not only possible but strongly encouraged by most practitioners. The synergy between 3BP and a ketogenic diet is well documented—ketosis further lowers glucose. Some protocols pair 3BP with hyperbaric oxygen therapy or other metabolic interventions for a one-two punch that attacks cancer from several angles. Timing matters: 3BP is often given during periods when blood glucose is at its lowest, maximizing tumor stress while protecting healthy cells. Tracking your labs—glucose, ketones, liver and kidney function—is critical for safety and to gauge effectiveness. Some patients keep a daily chart of symptoms, energy levels, and side effects to help their team tailor dosing and adjust supportive care.

If you're the kind of person who wants to know every detail—what's happening in your body, what to expect day by day—don't hesitate to ask your care team for as much information as possible. Request copies of your labs and scan results; keep a journal of your experiences during treatment. Not only does this help you feel more in control, but it can also provide valuable insights for others considering similar therapies.

Considering all this, 3BP stands as a beacon for those who feel out of options but aren't ready to give up, and for many facing late-stage cancers, it represents a real chance at stability, remission, or at least more time—often with a better quality of life than what aggressive chemo would allow. Remember, though, that any treatment comes with unknowns. Approach 3BP with curiosity and caution, ask lots of questions, and surround yourself with trusted support.

Hyperbaric Oxygen Therapy (HBOT)

The first time I heard about hyperbaric oxygen therapy, or HBOT, I pictured divers and scuba tanks. What I didn't expect was to find out just how much attention it's been getting in cancer circles—especially by people looking for gentler, more supportive options to add to their treatment plans. At its core, HBOT is about breathing pure oxygen while sitting or lying in a pressurized chamber. The basics sound simple, but the real magic happens on a cellular level. Under high pressure, your blood dissolves much more oxygen than it could at normal air pressure. This super-oxygenated blood travels throughout your body, reaching everywhere—even into tissues starved for air by swelling, tumors, or damage from surgery and radiation. For someone fighting cancer, that extra oxygen can be a powerful tool.

The science behind HBOT in the cancer setting starts with a key fact: most solid tumors grow in low-oxygen zones. Cancer cells thrive in these hypoxic pockets. In fact, a lack of oxygen is one way tumors dodge immune cells and resist chemo and radiation. They use these low-oxygen environments to hide and grow stronger. HBOT disrupts that hiding place. When you raise tissue oxygen levels, cancer cells lose one of their key advantages. Studies show that high oxygen levels can slow down cancer cell growth, make them less aggressive, and even trigger cell death in some cases. More importantly, healthy cells—unlike cancer—can adapt to extra oxygen, repair themselves faster, and recover from damage left by harsh treatments.

Now, when you pair HBOT with metabolic therapies like the ketogenic diet, the synergy can be even greater. Cancer cells—already stressed by low blood sugar levels and high ketones from keto—struggle to cope with a flood of oxygen. One study in mice found that combining a ketogenic diet with HBOT nearly doubled the lifespan of animals with aggressive brain tumors compared to either therapy alone. According to an article on PubMed Central, *"Ketogenic diet alone significantly decreased blood glucose, slowed tumor growth, and increased mean survival time by 56.7% in mice with systemic metastatic cancer. While HBO_2T alone did not influence cancer progression, combining the KD with HBO_2T elicited a significant decrease in blood glucose, tumor growth rate, and 77.9% increase in mean survival time compared to controls."*[10] The researchers believe that lowering glucose starves cancer cells, while HBOT delivers a knockout punch by ramping up oxidative stress inside the tumor. For people, this means the two therapies may work better together than apart. In practical terms, keto weakens the tumor's defenses, and HBOT finishes the job by making the environment toxic to cancer cells but safe for healthy ones.

If you're considering HBOT, you'll want to know what to expect. There are two main types of chambers: hard-shell chambers and soft-shell chambers. Hard-shell chambers can reach higher pressures (often 2–3 times atmospheric pressure) and deliver 100% oxygen, making them the gold standard for medical use. These are found in hospitals and specialized clinics. Soft-shell chambers, sometimes called "mild" HBOT chambers, use lower pressures (1.3–1.5 times atmospheric) and usually deliver room air or slightly enriched oxygen. They're more common in wellness centers or for home rental, but their cancer-fighting ability may not match the hard chambers. If you want the full therapeutic effect, find a certified clinic offering hard-shell HBOT with medical supervision.

Accessing HBOT can be easier said than done. In many countries, insurance will only pay for HBOT if you have one of a handful of approved conditions—like wound healing, carbon monoxide poisoning, or decompression sickness. Cancer isn't usually on that list. That means you may need to pay out of pocket or seek out integrative cancer clinics that offer HBOT specifically for adjunctive therapy. Always check credentials: look for clinics accredited by organizations such as the Undersea & Hyperbaric Medical Society (UHMS) or those with a licensed medical doctor present. Ask about their protocols for cancer patients, how many sessions they recommend, and what kind of chamber they use.

Safety should be top of mind. While HBOT is generally considered safe for most people, it's not risk-free. The most common side effects are mild—ear popping or pressure, sinus discomfort, and fatigue after a session. Rarely, people experience temporary changes in vision or mild oxygen toxicity if sessions are too long or pressure is too high. Serious risks—like lung problems or seizures—are very uncommon when treatment is done correctly in a certified setting. You should not use HBOT if you have certain lung conditions (like untreated pneumothorax), severe heart failure, or current ear infections. Always be honest about your health history and current medications when you talk to the clinic team.

Timing is everything if you want to integrate HBOT with other therapies. Many people schedule their HBOT sessions around chemotherapy cycles or after radiation to help speed up tissue repair and reduce inflammation. If you're also following a ketogenic diet or fasting protocol, talk with your care team about how to synchronize these strategies. Some clinics recommend arriving for HBOT sessions in a fasted state or with ketone levels elevated to maximize stress on the tumor. Others may schedule sessions right after chemo or immune therapy to help the body recover faster. Don't hesitate to ask for a written protocol or calendar so you can keep all your therapies organized.

If you're feeling overwhelmed by the options, it helps to break things down into steps. First, check if there's a certified HBOT clinic near you and book a consultation. Bring your latest scan results and a list of your current treatments. Ask about their experience with cancer patients specifically and request a tour of the chamber. If you move forward, track your energy levels, side effects, and any changes in symptoms. Some people notice better sleep or faster healing after just a few sessions; others may need weeks to see an impact.

In closing this chapter, remember that advanced metabolic and adjunctive therapies like HBOT offer another layer of hope and support. They're not magic bullets but can make your treatment plan stronger and kinder to your body. The next chapter will help you bridge these options with traditional care, showing how to create a team approach that respects both science and your personal choices.

Chapter 4
Fenbendazole — Fact, Protocol, and Practical Use

What Is Fenbendazole? Origins and Human Adaptation

Picture this: you're at your kitchen table, holding a packet with a dog on it, and wondering if it could help you fight cancer. This isn't where anyone expects to end up, yet many find themselves considering a pet medication, now central to discussions about hope, desperation, and science. Fenbendazole first entered my life through whispers in patient forums—perhaps you, too, heard about it from someone's story or via a late-night search or YouTube video. But before its use in cancer, let's clarify what fenbendazole is and why it exists.

Fenbendazole is a veterinary anti-parasitic drug, used for decades to treat intestinal worms and parasites in animals like dogs, cats, cattle, and horses. Part of the benzimidazole class, it disrupts microtubule formation in worm cells, preventing their growth and division. Approved by the FDA for animal use, fenbendazole quickly became a staple in veterinary medicine. You may have given it to your pets without a second thought. Vets appreciate its wide safety margin—animals rarely have serious side effects at correct doses.

So how did this dewormer make the leap to human cancer use? It didn't happen overnight or in research labs, but through stories of terminal cancer patients, like Joe Tippens, who experimented with fenbendazole after exhausting standard options. Tippens' widely shared personal success fueled curiosity and self-experimentation. Even before that, scientists noted that some benzimidazole drugs had anti-cancer properties in lab studies, interfering with cancer cell division as well as parasites. This made fenbendazole a candidate for drug repurposing—a movement searching for new uses for existing drugs.

Crucially, fenbendazole is not FDA-approved for human use anywhere. No pharmaceutical company officially produces it for people, no government regulates its effects in humans, and insurance won't cover complications. Use in people is considered "off-label" or "experimental," and most doctors won't recommend it due to a lack of approval. Fenbendazole is sold as powders, granules, or chewable tablets for animals, each with possibly different fillers or inactive ingredients—not all ideal or safe for people with allergies or sensitivities.

Regulatory standards for animal and human drugs differ significantly. Animal medications aren't held to the same purity or quality standards as human ones. While the active ingredient is usually present as labeled, quality and consistency can vary by brand or batch. Some products contain flavorings, binders, or preservatives for pet palatability and shelf life—not necessarily for human safety. This complicates sourcing: you must research brands, seek out certificates of analysis if available, and ensure you're not unknowingly consuming something harmful.

When it comes to safety, data is mixed but not alarming. Animal studies find that only extremely high doses of fenbendazole cause harm. Side effects in pets are rare and mild: occasional nausea, diarrhea, or tiredness if grossly overdosed. In humans, formal trials are lacking, but anecdotal reports and a few case series suggest side effects are uncommon at typical cancer protocol doses (usually 222 mg daily or less). Most reported effects are minor digestive issues or headaches; severe reactions are rare but not impossible. Importantly, no deaths have been directly attributed to fenbendazole in documented reports.

If you're considering fenbendazole for your cancer plan, here's a concise checklist:

Fenbendazole Safety Starter Checklist

- Check all ingredients; watch for artificial flavors or fillers.
- Avoid expired products; potency and safety can deteriorate.
- Start with a low dose if you have allergies or sensitivities.
- Monitor yourself for digestive changes (nausea, diarrhea).
- Don't start several new supplements or drugs at once; wait at least two weeks to start another new one, monitoring and noting any side effects.
- Tell someone you trust about your plan, and keep them updated on symptoms.
- Inform your oncologist if using alongside chemotherapy or immunotherapy—even if you anticipate disapproval.

Remember: hope should be grounded in informed, careful choices, not desperate gambles.

How Fenbendazole Works: Cancer Metabolism, Apoptosis, and Immune Effects

The big question most people have when they first hear about fenbendazole and cancer is simple: how does a dewormer even begin to affect a tumor? It's a fair question, and not one you'll often hear addressed by most oncologists. Fenbendazole's main action in animals is to disrupt microtubules—those tiny, tube-shaped proteins inside cells that act like scaffolding and highways for moving things around. For worms, this stops their cells from dividing and thriving, killing the parasite. But cancer cells also rely on microtubules to grow and multiply. When fenbendazole interferes with these structures, it throws a wrench in the rapid division that makes tumors so dangerous. Microtubule inhibition is a well-recognized strategy in cancer treatment; some chemotherapies like vincristine and paclitaxel work in similar ways. What's interesting about fenbendazole is that it seems to target these structures with less toxicity to normal cells, at least in lab settings.

It doesn't just stop cell division. Fenbendazole also messes with how cancer cells use sugar. You've probably heard the word "metabolism" thrown around, but in cancer, metabolism means the odd way tumors suck up glucose and ferment it for energy, even when oxygen is around. This is called aerobic glycolysis or the "Warburg effect." Cancer cells get hooked on sugar, and they are unable to live on ketones like healthy cells can. Fenbendazole throws off their sugar-burning machinery. Studies show it can lower the activity of key enzymes involved in glucose metabolism, starving the cancer cell from within. It's like suddenly slashing the fuel supply to a factory that never turns off its lights. For people trying to combine metabolic therapies like keto or carnivore diets with fenbendazole, this dual attack makes good sense—cut off glucose from outside and disrupt its use inside the cell.

Another big effect is apoptosis. This is science-speak for "programmed cell death"—the body's built-in way of telling sick or dangerous cells to self-destruct. Healthy bodies do this all the time, but cancer cells often escape this fate by disabling their own suicide mechanisms. Fenbendazole seems to help reactivate those signals. In laboratory tests, cancer cells exposed to the drug start showing classic signs of apoptosis: fragmentation, shrinkage, and even DNA breakdown. Think of apoptosis as an internal cleanup crew that's been locked out; fenbendazole might help unlock the doors.

The immune system gets pulled into the story too. Cancer is notorious for hiding from immune cells, creating a sort of cloaked fortress. Some early research suggests fenbendazole may help strip away that invisibility. It appears to increase expression of certain proteins on the outside of tumor cells, making them more visible to the immune system's surveillance. The body's natural killer cells and T-cells might have an easier time recognizing and attacking cancer when fenbendazole is in play. This area is still under investigation, but the idea of combining immune awakening with metabolic disruption is a big reason people are interested in "stacking" strategies that include this drug.

Lab and animal studies on fenbendazole's anti-cancer effects are promising but not perfect. There are documented cases where tumors in mice shrank or slowed down significantly after fenbendazole treatment. In petri dishes, human cancer cell lines—including those from lung, brain, and colon cancers—responded by stopping growth or dying off when exposed to the drug. These are controlled conditions, not the full complexity of a living human, but they're enough to justify more research and cautious hope. Some scientists have even tested fenbendazole alongside other treatments: combining it with chemo, radiation, or metabolic therapy often enhances the effects, at least in animals or lab cells.

Dr. Tom Rogers of Performance Medicine, also known as the "Common Sense MD," discusses, in a 17-minute video, how Fenbendazole (and also artemisinin) works against cancer[11].

Still, there are plenty of gaps in what we know. Researchers don't fully understand how fenbendazole gets absorbed and processed in the human body. There's little data on what happens when you take it for months instead of days, or how it interacts with other medications—especially chemo or immunotherapy drugs. We also don't know which cancers respond best or why some people see dramatic results while others see none. The lack of big clinical trials means most doctors remain cautious or dismissive, and patients are left sorting through scattered evidence and personal stories.

I'm not going to pretend the science is settled. There are real questions about dosing, long-term safety, and whether certain tumors adapt to outsmart fenbendazole over time. The research is ongoing, and as with any off-label or self-directed therapy, there's risk along with hope. For now, what's clear is that fenbendazole's story is more than just a viral anecdote—it's rooted in real biological mechanisms that deserve attention and careful study.

Documented Case Studies: Joe Tippens and Other Real-World Survivors

If you're like me, personal stories of cancer remission fill you with hope. It's important for us to remember that all of the stories and cases shared below are anecdotal and do not constitute scientific proof of causation or guaranteed outcomes.

When people first hear about fenbendazole, they usually want to know if anyone has actually beaten cancer with it. This is where the story of Joe Tippens comes in. His experience isn't just a rumor—it's one of the most widely known and discussed cases among people searching for alternative therapies. His cancer had spread to multiple areas of his body (neck, both lungs, stomach, bladder, liver, pancreas, and tailbone; dozens of tumors). Joe called a friend who was a veterinarian, and learned of a research scientist who was experimenting on cancers in mice and who, through trial and error, discovered that fenbendazole, a drug designed for dogs, healed the mice of the cancers. The research scientist, after being diagnosed with cancer and given three months to live, decided to try fenbendazole herself. Joe decided he had nothing to lose, and to try the drug alongside his prescribed treatments. He started taking 222 mg of fenbendazole daily (the dose found in one packet of Panacur C, a common dog dewormer), cycling three days on and four days off. After some research, Joe also added vitamin E, CBD oil, and curcumin to his regimen, but made it clear that fenbendazole was the main new variable.

Joe was one of 1,100 people involved in a cancer drug trial. He kept careful notes, but said nothing to his doctors about his protocol (he didn't want to be kicked out of the trial). and shared his progress online, making his story verifiable and open to scrutiny. By the end of 2017, his PET scan showed no evidence of active disease. A few months later, a second PET scan showed the same thing. Joe fessed up to his oncologist, who was shocked. Joe didn't hide behind anonymity; he provided scan results and allowed his medical records to be reviewed by others. He posted updates on his blog and social media so people could follow his case step by step, from diagnosis through remission. His experience became a beacon for others: not simply hope, but documented evidence that could be reviewed, questioned, and discussed.

I've included information on Joe Tippens' cancer support group in Resources. Joe's interview with Koco News 5 is in Resources.

Joe's case is not the only one out there. Other survivors have stepped forward with detailed records—some with lung cancer, others with brain, colon, or even breast cancer.

The following three case studies can be found at Karger.com[12].

Breast Cancer

An 83-years-old woman first faced breast cancer in 2009. Doctors removed both breasts, reconstructed them, and put her on medication to block estrogen (similar to restricting glucose), which had been fueling the cancer. She stopped taking those pills eventually but remained cancer-free for over a decade.

Then in October 2021, the cancer came back with a vengeance. This time it had spread throughout her body—to her liver, lungs, and spine. Tumors dotted her backbone from top to bottom, and the largest one in her lower spine was pressing into her spinal canal. Her liver was riddled with tumors, the biggest nearly three inches across. Six tumors grew in her lungs. The cancer had even blocked one of the tubes draining her liver, requiring doctors to insert a stent. Tests on fluid in her abdomen and tissue from her liver confirmed the cancer had spread everywhere. She was given a stage 4 diagnosis and placed in hospice care.

She refused chemotherapy and radiation. Instead, on November 22, 2021, she started taking 222 mg of fenbendazole daily on her own. A month later, she also began receiving fulvestrant injections, a hormone-blocking drug designed to starve the cancer. In January 2022, she agreed to targeted radiation on two particularly painful tumors in her spine. Those tumors vanished within days, taking her pain with them.

She continued taking fenbendazole every day for eight months. During that time, something remarkable happened. Her blood work improved dramatically—the cancer marker in her blood plummeted from 316 to 36.6. Her liver function, which had been compromised, returned to normal. By April 2022, a PET scan showed no signs of active cancer anywhere in her body. Two months later, in June 2022, doctors confirmed she showed NED. She was in complete remission.

All her treatments were stopped. Her doctors scheduled check-ups every few months to monitor her. Throughout everything, she kept taking her daily vitamin D and multivitamin. In July 2022, blood tests showed some temporary liver issues—whether from the fulvestrant, the fenbendazole, or both together, no one could say for certain. But her liver recovered within weeks, and her cancer markers kept falling to normal levels.

Follow-up scans continued to show no cancer. She experienced no harmful side effects from the fenbendazole at this dose. Nearly three years after entering remission, she remains cancer-free and still takes fenbendazole every day.

Prostate Cancer

At 75 years old, a man learned in December 2021 that his prostate cancer had returned and spread throughout his bones. He'd first been diagnosed a decade earlier and had surgery that seemed to work—his PSA levels, the blood test that tracks prostate cancer, stayed undetectable for a year and a half. But then the numbers started climbing again, signaling the cancer was back.

This time, scans revealed the cancer had spread aggressively. Tumors peppered his spine, pelvis, and the top of his right arm bone. His lymph nodes were swollen with cancer, including nodes near his aorta that hadn't been there before.

In December 2021, he started standard hormone-blocking therapy with Orgovix and Erleada, medications designed to cut off the testosterone that feeds prostate cancer. He also began taking Xgeva to protect his bones. On top of that, he assembled his own regimen of supplements and repurposed drugs: high-dose vitamin D with K2 and magnesium, melatonin, berberine, curcumin, artemisinin, cimetidine, and several other substances thought to fight cancer. He also started taking fenbendazole in December 2021, usually every day, at doses ranging from 222 to 444 mg, occasionally reducing the amount.

A year later, in December 2022, scans showed the bone tumors were shrinking. The cancer in his lymph nodes had completely disappeared. His PSA levels had dropped to undetectable and stayed there.

By January 2024, two years into treatment, imaging confirmed the bone lesions continued to shrink significantly. No new cancer sites appeared anywhere. In April 2024, a specialized scan showed that nearly all the bone lesions had no active cancer—they'd become just scar tissue in the bone. The kidney cyst they found showed no cancer activity, and his lymph nodes remained clear. His PSA stayed undetectable for over two years—below 0.05.

Throughout this entire time, his liver function remained normal with no side effects from the fenbendazole. After more than two years of steady improvement with no signs of progression, he remains in near-complete remission and continues taking fenbendazole along with his hormone therapy and bone-protecting medication.

Melanoma

In July 2020, a man discovered, at 63 years old, he had a growth on his hip. It was melanoma with a specific genetic mutation called BRAFV600, stage

IIIC. He started taking two targeted drugs, dabrafenib and trametinib, but had to stop after eight months because they were weakening his heart. Still, after a year of treatment, the cancer was gone. He stayed cancer-free for two years.

Then in December 2023, the melanoma came back. A biopsy found a small but aggressive tumor on his lower left abdomen. Scans revealed the cancer had spread throughout his body—nodules in the lining of his abdomen and behind it, spots in his stomach and intestines, lesions in his hip muscles, and a tumor in his lower spine. During these tests, doctors also discovered an unrelated cancer in his ureter—a different type of malignancy altogether.

His oncologist wanted to start immunotherapy with nivolumab (Opdivo) but recommended waiting until after more biopsies. During this waiting period in mid-December 2023, he started taking fenbendazole on his own, between 222 and 444 mg daily. The tumors in his ureter were blocking his ability to urinate, so he had surgery to remove them in mid-December.

A specialized blood test that tracks melanoma DNA fragments circulating in his bloodstream told the story clearly. On November 29, 2023, before starting fenbendazole, the reading was 123.37—high levels of cancer. Less than seven weeks later, on January 17, 2024, it had plummeted to 0.38. During those weeks, he'd also received two doses of nivolumab. By February 21, 2024, the test read zero—no detectable melanoma DNA in his blood.

At his February 2024 follow-up, scans and blood tests showed no evidence of disease anywhere. The melanoma was gone. Throughout his treatment, he took his regular supplements: vitamin C, an antibiotic called cephalexin, vitamin D, CoQ10, B12, and glutathione—the same routine he'd maintained before and after his cancer disappeared.

More than 11 months after being declared in remission, he remains melanoma-free.

The following case studies, and others, in which patients used repurposed drugs as adjunctive therapies, can be found at meakinmetaboliccare.com[13]

Not everyone sees dramatic results, but a small percentage report either stable disease or partial shrinkage—sometimes enough to delay further chemotherapy or allow for a break from harsh medications.

It's important to be honest about the range of outcomes. Some people experience amazing results, while others see no benefit at all. A few report mild digestive discomfort or headache, but most tolerate the drugs well. There are also stories of non-responders—people who use fenbendazole for months with no change in scan results or blood markers. Factors like lifestyle, cancer type, stage, concurrent treatments, and even genetics may influence how well someone responds. Sometimes, people combine fenbendazole with other therapies (metabolic diets, hyperbaric oxygen, supplements), so it's hard to say what made the difference. Still, the number of well-documented, publicly shared cases suggests that at least for some individuals, fenbendazole may play a role in controlling or even eliminating cancer.

Now, I know that not every case you read online should be believed. Credibility rests on certain pillars: clear documentation (medical scans, pathology reports, bloodwork), consistency in reporting (timelines that match up with medical records), and transparency about other treatments being used. A credible case study doesn't hide complications or setbacks; it includes them. Survivors who are willing to share their real names, provide access to medical records, and answer tough questions from both doctors and patients are the most trustworthy sources. The presence of a supportive medical team willing to monitor and report progress adds another layer of authenticity.

If you are considering fenbendazole, keep detailed notes and ask your medical team for copies of all scans and test results. Share your experience with others, but do so honestly—report both the good and the bad. The more transparent you are, the more helpful your story will be for someone else searching for hope. A confidential survey to share your cancer experience can be found at Cancer Support Community[14].

Lung Cancer

Lung cancer can be particularly challenging, but there are dozens of case studies of successful outcomes using fenbendazole, ivermectin, and mebendazole, along with the dosages used by weight, by The Medical Advisor on OneDayMD.com[15].

Many Different Cancer Types

There are hundreds of successful case reports of Stage 4 Cancer Remissions with Fenbendazole, Ivermectin and Mebendazole by The Medical Advisor on OneDayMD.com[16].

Step-by-Step Fenbendazole Dosing Protocols, Cycles, and "Stacking"

When you start considering fenbendazole as part of your cancer plan, the biggest questions are always about what to take, how much, and for how long. It can feel overwhelming, but there are some patterns and "recipes" that many people have used, most famously the Joe Tippens Protocol. Here's how it generally works: you take 222 mg of fenbendazole each day—usually measured as one packet of Panacur C dog dewormer. Most people manage it as three days on, four days off. This cycle repeats week after week, allowing the body a break and possibly reducing the risk of side effects. The idea behind cycling is to keep the cancer cells on their toes, never letting them fully adapt, while giving your organs a rest from constant processing. Some folks stick to this schedule for months at a time, while others adjust based on how they feel or what their scan results show.

Cycle variations pop up in almost every community discussion. Some users do five days on and two days off. A few even go with daily dosing for several weeks straight, followed by a full week of rest. There's no one-size-fits-all answer here. Your own body will guide you. If you notice fatigue, stomach upset, or odd symptoms, that's your cue to slow down or adjust. Some people working with open-minded doctors even get liver function tests every month or two just to be safe. No matter your schedule, consistency is key—missing doses here and there diminishes any potential effect, so set reminders or use a pill organizer to stay on track.

Stacking fenbendazole with other supplements is very common among self-directed users. Many follow Joe Tippens' original plan, which included fenbendazole (222 mg per day, three consecutive days per week) vitamin E (400-800 IU per day), CBD oil (25 mg daily), and curcumin (600 mg daily). Each plays a different role. Curcumin is believed to reduce inflammation and help sensitize cancer cells to treatment. CBD oil may support immune function and help with anxiety or sleep issues, while vitamin E potentially protects healthy cells from oxidative stress. People often add these supplements to their daily routine alongside fenbendazole, usually with food to minimize stomach aches. I recommend writing down what you start and when so you can trace back any unexpected side effects.

For a detailed breakdown of Joe Tippens' original protocol, plus a newer version enhanced by an oncologist, visit The Medical Advisor at OneDayMD.com[17].

Mistakes happen—especially when you're navigating this without formal medical supervision. Some people start too many new supplements at once and can't tell what's helping or causing trouble. Others use expired products or mix brands without checking for added fillers and flavorings that could cause allergic reactions. Skipping cycles or doubling up after a missed dose is another common pitfall—fenbendazole isn't like an antibiotic where you need to "catch up." If you miss a day, just pick up where you left off. Another mistake is not drinking enough water or neglecting to check for drug interactions if you're on other medications. Always read labels, and if something feels wrong—persistent nausea, yellowing skin, severe headache—pause the protocol and talk to your doctor.

Tracking your protocol makes an enormous difference. A simple notebook to record every date, dose, supplement, and any symptoms. You might prefer a spreadsheet or a medication tracking app on your phone—whatever works for you. Not only does this help you stay organized, but it also gives you a clear record to show your healthcare team or to share with others who might be following your path. Some people draw up color-coded calendars with cycles marked out or use sticker charts for motivation. Seeing your progress helps you stick with the plan and gives you something solid to look back on if you need to adjust.

Interactive Tool: Daily Protocol Tracker

Create a page or digital note titled "My Fenbendazole Protocol." List columns for Date, Dose (mg), Supplements Taken (CBD, curcumin, vitamin E), Symptoms/Notes, and Mood/Energy Level. Fill in each day before bed. Every two weeks, review your notes—look for patterns. Are there days when certain symptoms spike? Did changing your cycle affect your energy? Use these insights to fine-tune your approach and discuss any changes with your doctor or support group.

In wrapping up this chapter, remember that using fenbendazole is not about finding a miracle but about making informed choices and paying close attention to your body's signals. The protocols offer structure, but your real power lies in staying organized and honest with yourself. As we move forward, the next chapter will explore another repurposed drug—ivermectin—and how it fits into the bigger picture of adjunctive cancer care.

Chapter 5
Ivermectin — Mechanisms, Protocols, and Applications

Ivermectin's Anti-Cancer Mechanisms: Beyond Antiparasitics

Until a few years ago when ivermectin made news as being helpful to many people fighting Covid, most people—myself included—knew it only as a treatment for pets' heartworms or human lice and scabies. Its reputation as a simple antiparasitic means it's trusted for safety, inexpensive, and widely available. Yet, its background in veterinary and tropical disease medicine makes some patients and doctors question its place in cancer care. That skepticism is now shifting, as more people look into its potential anti-cancer uses with growing curiosity.

Avermectin (from which ivermectin is derived) was discovered in the late 1970s in Japan, derived from the soil microbe *Streptomyces avermitilis*. It earned its reputation by paralyzing parasites through disrupting their nervous systems—a breakthrough that won its inventors the Nobel Prize in Physiology or Medicine in 2015. Used for decades against river blindness and lymphatic filariasis, its safety in humans is notable: billions of doses administered globally have resulted in very few severe side effects when used properly. For those exploring alternative cancer treatments, this longstanding safety record is reassuring.

The story changed when studies found ivermectin affecting cancer cells in the lab. It didn't just kill parasites—it prompted tumor cells to self-destruct. This wasn't a fluke; research across many labs consistently found that ivermectin triggered apoptosis (programmed cell death) in cancer cells, leaving most healthy cells unharmed. Instead of bursting and causing inflammation, these dying cells dismantle themselves in a controlled way.

How does ivermectin do this? Cancer cells survive by overriding their natural death cues—dividing endlessly, ignoring signals to stop, and spreading (metastasizing) throughout the body. Ivermectin appears to reactivate those suppressed cell-death pathways, especially within the mitochondria (the cell's energy center). By disrupting the mitochondrial function of cancer cells it initiates apoptosis.

Besides inducing apoptosis, ivermectin inhibits cancer proliferation—put simply, it slows cancer's rapid, unchecked division. The drug interferes with the cell cycle checkpoints that act as quality control for cell division. By restoring these checkpoints, it either puts cancer cells into arrest or nudges them to self-destruct instead of multiply.

Ivermectin also inhibits metastasis—the spreading of cancer. Lab and animal studies show that it blocks enzymes needed for cancer to invade new tissues, and suppresses proteins responsible for cell migration and adhesion, making it more difficult for tumors to spread.

Another intriguing aspect is its effect on cancer stem cells, thought to drive resistance and relapse. These hard-to-kill cells often survive treatment and spark new tumors later. Some early evidence suggests ivermectin targets these cells, potentially reducing recurrence rates. Research is early, but this holds promise for relapse prevention.

Ivermectin's potential crosses many cancer types. Laboratory work has tested it on breast, colon, ovarian, prostate, lung, leukemia, brain (glioblastoma), melanoma, and more. Across these, it consistently induced apoptosis, slowed growth, suppressed spread, and impaired cancer stem cell functions. Some studies combined it with standard therapies like chemotherapy or radiation, observing enhanced effects.

Human data remains limited but is building. A few published case series and early-phase clinical trials report encouraging responses (partial remissions or stable disease) in patients with advanced cancers like stomach, colon, breast, and even drug-resistant leukemia when ivermectin was added to standard treatments. These are individual cases, not definitive proof, but the results are enough to fuel more research.

Most supporting research is preclinical (in test tubes and animals), not from large, controlled human trials. Early clinical reports are intriguing but insufficient to define which cancer types respond best or to establish standard protocols. Progress is slow mainly because, as a generic and inexpensive drug, ivermectin isn't attractive to big pharmaceutical companies, leaving most ongoing research to be academic or crowdfunded.

To simplify: ivermectin pushes cancer cells toward programmed death, slows their growth, blocks the spread, and might reduce recurrence by targeting cancer stem cells. These effects are strong enough in preclinical studies that continued research and cautious clinical interest are warranted.

Interactive: Quick "Ivermectin Mechanisms" Case Reflection

List three questions about ivermectin and your (or your loved one's) specific cancer type. For instance: Could blocking metastasis help our case? Would combining ivermectin with current therapy be worth discussing? Take these questions to your next medical appointment or support group.

Because results often differ between lab experiments and real-world outcomes, it's vital to proceed carefully. There are still uncertainties:

variations in dosing protocols across studies, differences in cancer subtype responses, and unknown long-term safety with extended or higher-dosage use. That said, traditional use supports ivermectin's low toxicity at standard doses, though off-label or prolonged cancer uses require closer monitoring.

Facing uncertainty in your cancer journey is difficult, especially when searching for options now, not later. But informed, clear-eyed conversations—factoring in both potential benefits and what hasn't yet been proven—leave you better positioned than simply following unverified reports online.

Cancer care almost always means balancing scientific evidence with lived experience, caution with hope. Ivermectin exemplifies this tension: a safe, familiar, generic drug now repurposed in research for conditions far beyond its original antiparasitic use. Interest is especially high among those seeking gentler adjuncts to conventional treatment or who feel out of options.

Researchers continue tracking ivermectin responses across many cancers, including hard-to-treat brain tumors (where crossing the blood-brain barrier is key), and others like breast, prostate, lung, colon, leukemia, and lymphoma. The excitement isn't just in isolated anecdotes but in a repeated pattern: this old drug can trigger cell death in cancers that resist usual therapies.

Mainstream oncology doesn't yet recommend ivermectin for routine cancer use, but interest is rising alongside patient stories and new lab results indicating anti-cancer actions that are distinct from its antiparasitic origins. It's a potent example of medical discovery: sometimes, old drugs provide new answers, often hiding in unexpected places.

Understanding the mechanisms doesn't guarantee success for any individual, but it arms you with knowledge for more productive treatment discussions. As research grows, so will clarity about ivermectin's role—likely moving from faint hope to a better-defined place in comprehensive cancer care.

Human Dosing Protocols for Ivermectin: Safety and Scheduling

When exploring ivermectin for cancer, the lack of standardized dosing is a major hurdle. No clear prescription exists; instead, dosing recommendations are drawn from clinical practice, patient reports, and decades of use for other diseases. Generally, protocols circulating online commonly suggest 0.2–0.4 mg per kilogram of body weight per dose. For a 154 lb. (70 kg) adult, this is 14–28 mg per dose. These values are adapted from antiparasitic treatments and observed anti-cancer effects in lab and animal studies, with a handful of clinicians supervising off-label use. Most case reports and anecdotes stay within this 0.4 mg/kg threshold to maintain safety, especially for prolonged regimens.

Some protocols advise taking the dose all at once, while others split it into two daily doses. There's no firm evidence favoring one method over the other—as long as you hit the total daily target for your weight. Many start at 0.2 mg/kg for a week or two, then increase if tolerated, which helps reduce side effects, especially for sensitive individuals or those on other medications.

Scheduling varies, too. Protocols range from continuous daily dosing to cyclic schedules (e.g., five days on, two days off; three weeks on, one week off). Cycling is adapted from chemotherapy protocols to allow your liver and kidneys a rest, helpful if you're on other drugs. Those experiencing nausea or fatigue from cancer treatments may prefer these scheduled breaks. Some clinicians recommend pausing ivermectin during episodes of low white blood cells or intensive chemo, then resuming afterward. There's no universal schedule—what counts is listening to your body and tracking weekly responses.

While concerns about interactions with chemo, immunotherapy, or targeted therapies persist, current evidence suggests ivermectin (in these doses) is generally safe to use alongside standard treatments, with careful monitoring. Some oncologists are open to combining ("stacking") ivermectin during or between chemo cycles; others may be hesitant. Share your plans with your doctor if possible. While there are no major reports of harm from combining ivermectin with other cancer treatments at the discussed doses, proceed with caution, listen to your body, and document everything.

The Medical Advisor at OneDayMD.com has handy charts for assisting with ivermectin dosage[18].

Safety remains a top concern with off-label use, especially for cancer. Billions tolerate short-term ivermectin well, but longer-term or high-dose use requires care. Most side effects—nausea, diarrhea, dizziness, rash, metallic taste—are mild. Rarely, headaches or blurred vision appear and usually resolve if dosing stops or decreases. Severe reactions (allergies, liver toxicity) are rare but possible, especially with pre-existing liver disease. Basic blood tests—liver enzymes (ALT, AST), kidney function (creatinine, BUN), and CBC—are recommended before starting, then every 4–8 weeks if used over a month. Stop and consult a doctor immediately if you have marked changes in labs or develop jaundice.

Practical organization tools simplify adherence. Use pill organizers and daily alarms, and set a consistent time to take your dose with food to aid absorption and reduce GI upset. Track doses and symptoms in a notebook or app and clearly mark cycling schedules (e.g., five on/two off) on a calendar. Summarize your whole regimen on one page (doses, timing, notes), share it with a trusted friend or caregiver, and take it to medical appointments—helpful for spotting missed doses or changes.

Community support from online groups or forums can help with doubts or side effect management, but always remember that individual responses vary.

For those unable to swallow pills, ivermectin comes as tablets, oral solutions, and compounded forms (from pharmacies). Tablets offer the easiest dosing accuracy. Since ivermectin for humans is available, avoid veterinary formulations, as they may contain unsafe additives. Opt for pharmaceutical-grade sources and check quality assurances.

Adherence means more than taking pills; it requires ongoing self-monitoring. If you miss a dose, don't double up—just resume the schedule. New or worsening symptoms, especially neurological ones, warrant suspending the protocol and seeking medical advice (these are rare but serious).

Adjust ivermectin timing around your lifestyle. Some experience mild fatigue or digestive symptoms, prompting tweaks in meal or activity timing. If using supplements (e.g., curcumin, vitamin D, omega-3s), separate them from ivermectin by a couple of hours to minimize unknown interactions.

If using alongside chemotherapy, align ivermectin doses with periods when your GI tract is less aggravated, or use it during chemo "off" weeks. Some continue through the cycle, but careful monitoring is always a good idea.

Lab checks are your main way to prevent or catch side effects early. Track baseline labs before starting and repeat them monthly or as advised, especially if you have rare cancers or take other strong medicines.

Cost is another advantage—Ivermectin is far cheaper than most cancer drugs or supplements and widely available as generics, though supply disruptions happen. Compounding pharmacies can help, if standard supplies are unavailable, with a doctor's prescription.

In summary, a successful ivermectin protocol means starting with a weight-based dose (usually 0.2–0.4 mg/kg), choosing a practical dosing schedule, and staying vigilant about recording your responses.

Most importantly, you aren't alone. Many are experimenting and sharing insights. Reach out to support groups, informed clinicians, or others on the same journey if you need guidance.

Practical Adherence Checklist

- Calculate dose by weight (0.2–0.4 mg/kg)
- Select daily or cyclic schedule; mark off days
- Take with food to ease stomach issues

- Use a pill organizer and set alarms
- Track doses and side effects
- Review the plan weekly
- Repeat lab work every 4–8 weeks (liver, kidney, CBC)
- Inform your care team or a trusted friend
- Buy only from reputable, human pharmacies
- Pause and get help if new symptoms appear

Ivermectin protocols demand careful organization and awareness, but are manageable with a steady approach. Make adjustments as needed and focus on what works for you—aiming for the best chance at health.

The next chapter explores repurposed drugs in combination with metabolic therapies, dietary strategies, and holistic supports, building a complete approach addressing body, mind, and spirit.

Chapter 6
Comparing and Combining Repurposed Drugs

Fenbendazole vs. Ivermectin: Synergy and Differences

You might find yourself holding two different bottles—one labeled for dogs, another for livestock or humans—wondering which could actually make a dent in something as relentless as cancer. Maybe you've read a dozen stories online about people mixing and matching these drugs in search of an edge. It's normal to feel both hopeful and overwhelmed. There's no shame in bouncing between curiosity and caution, especially with so much conflicting advice floating around. Many people wonder whether fenbendazole or ivermectin is "the one." The truth is, both have their strengths and quirks. The real power, though, comes from understanding how they overlap, where they split off, and whether combining them makes sense for you.

At first glance, fenbendazole and ivermectin seem like odd candidates for cancer care. They weren't designed for humans, let alone as weapons against tumors. Yet, here they are, at the center of a movement that's as grassroots as it is scientific. Fenbendazole started as a worm killer for pets. Ivermectin found its fame fighting river blindness and scabies in people across the world. Over time, researchers noticed something curious: both drugs interfere with the machinery that keeps cancer cells alive, but they go about it in different ways. This means you're not just choosing between two pills—you're deciding between two strategies that attack cancer from unique angles, and sometimes those approaches complement each other.

Digging into the science, you see that fenbendazole and ivermectin share some territory when it comes to how they work. Both disrupt microtubules—tiny scaffolding inside cells that help them divide and multiply. Cancer cells are obsessed with division; they need these microtubules to keep their chaotic growth going. When you take fenbendazole, you're jamming up the assembly lines that let tumors clone themselves. Ivermectin also meddles with microtubules to some extent, but its real tricks show up elsewhere. It interferes with signaling pathways that cancer cells use to dodge death, especially those involving mitochondria (the cell's powerhouses). By doing so, ivermectin pushes cancer cells toward apoptosis—without causing the messy inflammation that comes from uncontrolled cell death.

There's more overlap: both drugs shut down certain metabolic functions unique to cancer cells. Tumors often display what's called the "Warburg effect"—they gorge on glucose and rely on fermentation even when oxygen is plentiful. Fenbendazole tampers with enzymes that help cancer cells burn sugar, starving them from the inside out. Ivermectin, while not a metabolic drug in the classic sense, also disrupts cellular energy production by messing with mitochondrial function. So you get a kind of double whammy: both drugs create an environment where cancer finds it harder to fuel its growth.

Yet for all their similarities, fenbendazole and ivermectin diverge in important ways. Fenbendazole's main claim to fame is interfering with microtubule assembly and targeting glucose metabolism. It's like sabotaging the roads and fuel supply at the same time. Ivermectin's reach is broader—it not only disrupts some microtubules but also blocks communication signals between cancer cells and their environment, suppresses the spread of tumors (metastasis), and may even make cancer stem cells—the seeds of recurrence—less likely to survive. Some research suggests ivermectin can also enhance immune detection of tumors, peeling away their disguises so the body's natural defenses have a fighting chance.

What happens when you combine these two? The idea of synergy—the whole being greater than the sum of its parts—comes up a lot in cancer treatment circles. The hope is that using both drugs together could hit cancer on multiple fronts at once: preventing division, disrupting metabolism, triggering cell death, and waking up the immune system. In theory, this cocktail could make it much harder for a tumor to adapt or develop resistance. Laboratory studies support this logic: using drugs with complementary mechanisms can increase cancer cell kill rates compared to single agents alone. Some patients have reported better outcomes when stacking fenbendazole with ivermectin than with either one solo; they describe tumor shrinkage or longer periods of stability on scans. However, these reports are mostly anecdotal—shared in forums or self-published logs—large clinical trials are still missing.

Safety is where things get personal. Both drugs have long histories in animals and, in ivermectin's case, billions of human doses for other diseases. Fenbendazole rarely causes serious side effects in either pets or people using typical protocols; mild digestive upset or headache are the most common issues. Ivermectin is generally safe at standard doses but can cause dizziness, rash, or stomach discomfort in some people. Most reactions go away if you lower the dose or take a break. The risk profile changes if you combine them—mainly because your liver and kidneys need to process both together. If you already have organ stress from chemo or other medications, adding more can increase your risk of side effects or drug interactions.

That's why sequencing or stacking should be tailored to your own health situation and goals. Some choose to try fenbendazole for a few months while monitoring symptoms and blood work closely before adding ivermectin. Others alternate weeks or cycle one drug for several days and then switch to the other. There's no official playbook—most protocols are adapted from what patients report works best for their bodies and lifestyles.

If you're deciding between these agents or thinking about using both, here's a stepwise approach that has helped others:

First, get a clear picture of your current health status: liver and kidney function tests, any allergies or past drug reactions, what standard treatments you're on now (chemo, immunotherapy, targeted therapies), and your baseline energy level. This isn't just about safety—it helps you notice real changes once you start.

Next, choose one agent to begin with—usually fenbendazole if you're looking for metabolic disruption first, or ivermectin if your priority is immune modulation or addressing metastatic spread. Start at the lowest recommended dose: 222 mg daily for fenbendazole (cycled three days on/four days off), or 0.2–0.4 mg/kg for ivermectin (daily or cyclic). Stick with this for two to four weeks while tracking side effects and checking labs.

If tolerated well and you're not seeing negative trends in your labs or symptoms, consider introducing the second agent—either by overlapping cycles (for example, fenbendazole on Monday-Wednesday and ivermectin on Thursday-Saturday), or by extending your cycle (one week on fenbendazole followed by one week on ivermectin). Pay close attention to how you feel each day, and don't hesitate to pause if anything feels off.

Some people find they tolerate both drugs well together at lower doses than when taken alone—this is where synergy might show up without increasing toxicity. For example, you might use fenbendazole at 150 mg daily instead of 222 mg when taking it alongside ivermectin at 0.2 mg/kg every other day.

Monitoring is everything here. Repeat liver and kidney tests every month; check in with your doctor or an integrative practitioner if possible—even if they aren't fully on board with your plan, they can help spot issues early. Keep a journal of doses taken, days off, side effects noticed (from mild nausea to rashes or unusual fatigue), energy levels, and any new symptoms. I know I keep saying this—it's important.

There are special considerations if you're using other supplements or medications. Both drugs can interact with substances metabolized by the liver's cytochrome P450 system—a kind of internal filter for breaking down chemicals. If you're taking medications like statins, antifungals, antibiotics, or immune modulators, double-check compatibility with a pharmacist or knowledgeable integrative doctor.

Choosing between fenbendazole and ivermectin involves figuring out which fits your biology and goals best at this moment. If your main concern is rapid tumor growth that doesn't respond to standard therapy, stacking might offer more pressure on multiple weak spots in the cancer's armor. If you have minimal disease left but want to avoid recurrence, alternating cycles could balance effectiveness with safety.

For people who feel especially sensitive to medications or who have struggled with side effects before, starting slow and low makes sense; it's not a race. For those whose cancers seem aggressive or resistant, combining sooner rather than later can feel urgent—but always weigh potential benefits against risks unique to your situation.

Interactive: Protocol Reflection & Tracking Tool

Set up a simple tracking chart titled "My Repurposed Drug Protocol." Down the left side list days of the week; across the top make columns for "Fenbendazole Dose," "Ivermectin Dose," "Other Meds/Supps," "Energy Level," "Side Effects," "Mood," and "Notes." Each evening before bed, fill in your doses and reflect on how you felt—physically and emotionally—that day. Every Sunday night, review your notes for trends: Did new side effects crop up after adding a drug? Did fatigue improve with dose adjustments? Share this log with your support team for feedback.

In this sea of options—where hope meets uncertainty—remember that protocols are tools to be adjusted rather than rules set in stone. Listen to your own body above all else. Protocols online are starting points; your experience will guide the real journey forward. Stay connected to others who truly listen without judgment—patients sharing their stories online are often more honest than any product insert or scientific review.

If you ever feel stuck choosing what's next—or just scared about making the wrong call—step back and check in with your values: Do you want more control? Fewer side effects? A shot at slowing things down? There's no single right answer here. Your life is not an experiment; it's precious ground for making choices that fit who you are right now.

The science keeps evolving—and so will these protocols—but what will always matter most is that you feel informed enough to steer your care with confidence and support around you every step of the way.

Other Promising Repurposed Drugs

In my search for answers, I quickly realized that fenbendazole and ivermectin are just two names in a long and growing list of repurposed drugs people are exploring for cancer. It wasn't long before I stumbled onto **mebendazole**. If you've ever dealt with pinworms as a parent or patient, you might recognize it as that old standby, the chewable tablet for kids. It's another benzimidazole, like fenbendazole, but approved for human use in many countries and available in pharmacies. What caught my attention was how it attacks cancer cells using a similar playbook—disrupting microtubules to stop cell division, slowing tumor growth. But it also seems to have unique effects, like reducing blood supply to tumors by blocking angiogenesis and helping the immune system spot abnormal cells. Lab research and early case reports show promise for brain tumors, colon cancer, and even melanoma. While not a magic bullet, the evidence is strong enough that some doctors in Europe are running pilot studies for tough-to-treat cancers.

Dosing mebendazole for cancer is something people often figure out by pulling together bits and pieces from research papers and patient experience. Most protocols use 100-200 mg, two or three times a day, with or without food. Some patients pulse it—taking it for three weeks followed by a break—while others stay on lower doses for longer stretches. It's generally well-tolerated, with rare side effects like mild stomach upset or rash. Since it's already used in children, its safety profile is reassuring to many adults. However, long-term use, especially at higher doses, may affect liver enzymes or cause mild bone marrow suppression, so regular bloodwork is important. For those who can't get fenbendazole or prefer a medication already approved for humans, mebendazole feels less risky, and you don't have to worry as much about what else is in the pill besides the active ingredient. This makes it a practical choice for people nervous about veterinary drugs or those with allergies to animal flavorings and dyes.

As discussed previously, it's important to remember that all of the stories and cases shared below are anecdotal and do not constitute scientific proof of causation or guaranteed outcomes.

Case Study: Brain Cancer (Glioblastoma)

On March 31, 2023, a 68-year old man sought medical attention for weakness in his right hand. Imaging revealed a brain mass: glioblastoma. Prognosis was 3-4 months without treatment; up to two years with treatment.

He underwent two extensive laser surgeries which removed as much of the tumor as possible, and started on standard cancer treatments (chemo and radiation).

Meanwhile, the patient's wife discovered a book entitled "Keto for Cancer" by Miriam Kalamian. They arranged a consultation with the author, and the wife meticulously prepared his keto meals at home.

Under the direction of the Meakin Clinic, the patient began using Doxycycline, Metformin, Atorvastatin, and Mebendazole, and supplemented Vitamin D3, Vitamin K2, Omega-3 Fish Oils (2000 mg/day), and Melatonin(10-20 mg/day). He also pulsed with Hyperbaric Oxygen Therapy (HBOT). All this was integrated with his standard cancer treatments. With physical therapy, he regained his ability to walk without a wheelchair or cane, used previously.

By the end of July, 2023, the outcome was NED, as evidenced by an MRI.

Case Study: Colon Cancer Stage IIIb:

In February 2018, a 55-year old man discovered through a colonoscopy that he had adenocarcinoma with the involvement of ten lymph nodes. He underwent surgery and a 6-month course of oral chemotherapy.

In 2019, he began the repurposed drugs doxycycline, metformin, atorvastatin, and mebendazole. Supplements included calcium, zinc, polyphenol, Mega Free tea extract, vitamin D3 + K2, liver GI detox, lion's mane for cognition, cinnamon, Circuit Eval 400, Coriolus versicolor, Ultimate Omega D3, and melatonin. Infrared sauna was also used in his treatment plan.

He ate a Mediterranean-inspired diet with plenty of healthy oils, vegetables, moderate meat and fruit, and low in sugar. His overall wellness practices included 1.5 hours of exercise daily (resistance training, cardio, aerobics, and balance work). As of the case writing (August 2024) he had NED for six years.

Case Study: Pancreatic Cancer 1:

In May of 2019, a 73-year old female, who was in remission from a 2015 diagnosis of breast cancer, was diagnosed with pancreatic cancer, including 1 of 6 lymph nodes tested. She underwent twelve sessions of chemotherapy, and one month of radiation therapy, followed by Whipple Surgery in January 2020, in which the head of the pancreas, gallbladder, common bile duct, and duodenum were removed.

She used the repurposed drugs Metformin, Doxycycline, Atorvastatin, and Mebendazole, along with a Mediterranean diet of proteins, vegetables, and fruits but low in sugar, with five one-hour exercise sessions weekly, and HBOT.

As of the writing of this case report (August 2024), she has survived over four years since her original diagnosis. (According to Meakin Clinic, *"The*

5-year survival rate for stage 4 pancreatic cancer is notably low, around 1-3%.")

Case Study: Pancreatic Cancer 2:

In October 2019, a 78-year old male was diagnosed with pancreatic cancer, and underwent surgery in October and November of that year. In January 2020, he began chemotherapy, followed by one month of radiation.

He used the adjunctive therapies of high-dose Vitamin-C injections, and pulsing metabolic therapy. He used the repurposed drugs Metformin, Doxycycline, Atorvastatin, Mebendazole, and the supplements Vitamin D3, Vitamin K2, Omega-3 Fish Oils, Melatonin.

His diet consisted of lots of salmon and salads, and other clean meats, with low sugar.

He experienced a brief recurrence in May 2020, but has shown NED since then.

One thing that struck me as I was reading through the case reports above, and many others, is that they have a common thread: a clean, low-carb diet as part of an overall wellness program. I believe that diet and lifestyle choices are of utmost importance.

Nitazoxanide is another drug that quietly emerged from the world of infectious disease. Originally prescribed for parasitic and viral infections—think giardia, cryptosporidium, or even certain flus—it works by interfering with how pathogens replicate. Researchers noticed it also blocks certain metabolic pathways in cancer cells, including the use of glucose and lactic acid, and disrupts the signals that let tumors evade the immune system. It's especially interesting because it reaches high concentrations in tissues where some cancers like to hide, including the liver and colon. Some early-stage clinical trials are now testing nitazoxanide for pancreatic cancer and colorectal cancer, often in combination with chemotherapy or immune therapies. The results are still rolling in, but suggest that adding nitazoxanide can help shrink tumors or stabilize disease where standard treatments alone fall short.

When it comes to dosing nitazoxanide, most protocols use 500 mg twice a day, usually with food to avoid stomach irritation. This is the same dose used in infectious disease, so there's plenty of safety data. Common side effects include nausea or mild diarrhea, but these tend to be short-lived. In rare cases, people experience headaches or yellowing of the skin, so liver function monitoring is wise for long-term use. One plus is that nitazoxanide doesn't seem to interact much with other meds, making it less complicated to combine with standard cancer drugs or supplements. You can get it as a tablet or suspension, and it's available through regular pharmacies in most countries, which takes away some sourcing anxiety.

Beyond the more familiar drugs, other antihelmintics and anti-infectives keep popping up in forums and emerging research. **Albendazole** is one example; while structurally similar to mebendazole and fenbendazole, it appears to cross into the brain a bit more easily, making it a point of interest for brain tumors and metastases. The downside is that it can be rougher on the liver and bone marrow, so it's used less often outside of clinical trials or highly supervised protocols. Then there's **pyrvinium pamoate**, a bright red medicine once used for pinworms in children. Now, scientists are investigating it for its ability to disrupt cancer cell metabolism and block the growth of stem-like tumor cells. Most of this work is lab-based, though a few compassionate use cases are filtering into the literature.

Some anti-infectives from other drug classes have also shown anti-cancer effects. **Doxycycline**, a common antibiotic for acne or respiratory infections, can shut down certain enzymes that help cancer spread and may even sensitize tumors to chemo or radiation. **Metronidazole**, often known as Flagyl, has shown activity in slowing tumor growth by changing the low-oxygen environments inside solid cancers. These drugs aren't at the top of most alternative protocols, but for people who have exhausted other options or need something that crosses into the brain or bone, they're worth a conversation with an integrative physician.

Each repurposed drug comes with its own set of strengths and risks. Mebendazole's human approval and gentle side effect profile make it comfortable for long-term use or for those with sensitivities to additives.

Nitazoxanide offers versatility, as it seems to hit both cancer metabolism and immune evasion. It's easy to access and stack with other therapies. Albendazole is more potent but harder on the body; routine blood tests are a must if you try it. Pyrvinium pamoate is still experimental and challenging to source outside specific programs. Antibiotics like doxycycline or metronidazole are familiar to most people, but long-term use can affect gut health or cause yeast overgrowth, so probiotics or gut support may be needed.

Access challenges are real. Some drugs, like mebendazole and nitazoxanide, are prescription-only in many countries. If your doctor is open-minded or you have a cooperative pharmacist, this helps. Others may only be available from online pharmacies or require travel to countries where regulations are looser. Veterinary versions might be tempting for cost or convenience, but always check the fillers and manufacturing standards—your health is too precious to gamble on unknowns.

If You're Feeling Overwhelmed, Start Here

A cancer diagnosis can make every option feel urgent and confusing. If the information in this book feels like too much at once, pause. You do not need to implement everything.

Begin with these four foundational steps:

1. Stabilize your metabolic baseline. Focus first on reducing excess sugar intake and improving dietary quality. Then consider a gradual transition toward a lower-carbohydrate or ketogenic approach under supervision.

2. Establish monitoring. Before adding any new therapies, obtain baseline labs (liver enzymes, kidney function, blood counts). Start tracking symptoms and energy levels.

3. Add only one change at a time. Whether it's a repurposed drug, supplement, fasting window, or HBOT session—introduce one variable and observe.

4. Reassess regularly. Every 4–8 weeks, evaluate: labs, symptoms, tolerance, and overall well-being. Adjust thoughtfully.

You do not need a perfect protocol. You need a monitored, adaptable plan.

Minimal Starting Path:

- Improve diet quality
- Monitor labs
- Discuss options with physician
- Avoid stacking multiple new agents at once

Personalizing Your Protocol

Integrating these drugs into your protocol requires thoughtful planning. You want to avoid doubling up on similar mechanisms unless you have clinical guidance. For example, mebendazole and fenbendazole both disrupt microtubules; stacking them might not add much benefit but could increase liver strain. Instead, many people "stack" drugs with complementary actions—such as combining a microtubule disruptor like mebendazole with a metabolic agent like nitazoxanide or an immune modulator like ivermectin. The goal is to hit the cancer from several sides without overwhelming your body's ability to process the drugs.

Sample stacks often look like this: mebendazole 100 mg twice daily, nitazoxanide 500 mg twice daily, plus a lower dose of ivermectin every other day. Or, for someone focused on brain tumors, albendazole might replace mebendazole, but with more frequent blood tests. Supplements like curcumin (for inflammation) or melatonin (for sleep and immune support), or glycine (for sleep, antioxidant activity and liver detox) are sometimes added, but it's wise to introduce only one new thing at a time so you can pinpoint any problems. Always track your doses, side effects, energy, and mood. A simple notebook or spreadsheet can make a world of difference in understanding what's helping—or what's not.

If you're combining repurposed drugs with chemotherapy or radiation, timing matters. Some protocols recommend taking these meds during chemo "off weeks" to give your body a break and avoid unexpected interactions. Others suggest low daily doses throughout treatment for ongoing metabolic pressure. No matter what you choose, check drug interaction databases or consult a pharmacist familiar with oncology. Even safe-seeming meds can amplify side effects of standard treatments.

A big part of integrating repurposed drugs is honest communication—with your medical team if possible, but also with yourself and someone you trust. If you feel unsure, start slow. Add one drug at a time, monitor labs and symptoms, and don't hesitate to pause if anything feels off. Share your protocol with your partner or a close friend; a second set of eyes can spot changes you might miss.

Reflection Prompt: Building Your Stack

Take a moment to map out what you're using now—include prescription drugs, supplements, and any repurposed agents under consideration. On a fresh page or spreadsheet, write down the purpose of each: is it for metabolism, immune support, microtubule disruption, or something else? Are there overlaps? Where could you simplify? Where might you add something new? Jot down any questions you'd like to ask your doctor or pharmacist. Review this list weekly as you adjust your protocol.

In this world of repurposed drugs, flexibility is your ally. Protocols can—and frankly should—change as you gather new information and experience how your body responds. There's no one-size-fits-all stack. What matters most is learning to listen closely: to your own body, to honest reports from others, and to the evolving science that continues to surprise us all.

Bringing it all together, repurposed drugs like mebendazole, nitazoxanide, albendazole, pyrvinium pamoate, and even familiar antibiotics offer new possibilities for those seeking options beyond standard cancer care. Each has unique strengths and challenges, and integrating them thoughtfully can open doors that once seemed closed. The next chapter explores how to build a truly integrative approach—combining the best of alternative and conventional medicine while protecting your safety and hope along the way.

Repurposed Agents at a Glance

Mechanism Overview: Repurposed Agents at a Glance

AGENT	PRIMARY ACTION	GLUCOSE TARGETING	GLUTAMINE IMPACT	IMMUNE MODULATION	KEY MONITORING
FENBENDAZOLE	Microtubule disruption; possible metabolic stress	Indirect	Possible indirect	Mild	Liver enzymes
MEBENDAZOLE	Microtubule disruption; anti-angiogenic effects	Indirect	Some research support	Mild	Liver function, CBC
IVERMECTIN	Wnt/β-catenin modulation; ion channel effects	Indirect	No direct evidence	Yes	Neurologic symptoms
NITAZOXANIDE	Mitochondrial metabolism interference	Yes	Possible indirect	Yes	Liver enzymes
ALBENDAZOLE	Microtubule disruption; better CNS penetration	Indirect	Unclear	Mild	Liver function, CBC
DOXYCYCLINE	Mitochondrial protein synthesis inhibition	Indirect	No direct	Mild	GI tolerance
METRONIDAZOLE	Hypoxia modulation	Indirect	No direct	Minimal	Neurologic symptoms
3-BROMOPYRUVATE (3BP)*	Glycolysis inhibition	Direct	No	No	Strict clinical supervision

Chapter 7
Sourcing Repurposed Drugs Safely

Universal Principles for Vetting Suppliers

Staring at a website peddling alternative cancer drugs, I felt my stomach twist. I wondered if what I was seeing was real or dangerous. You might know the feeling—scrolling through endless products and promises, unsure if you'll be scammed or harmed. Thankfully, you can protect yourself using a handful of universal principles to vet any supplier.

First, look for transparency. Trustworthy suppliers reveal product origins, list all active and inactive ingredients, and provide batch numbers for traceability. If important details are missing or hard to find, take it as a red flag. Consistent branding, clear labeling, and accessible customer support also indicate reliability.

Next, always check for Certificates of Analysis (COA). This document confirms an independent lab has tested the product for identity, purity, and contaminants. Even reputable veterinary medicines have COAs. No COA? Move on—the risks aren't worth it. You want proof to back up claims, not empty assurances. **Another principle: look for genuine reviews with detailed stories rather than just five-star ratings.** If there are repeated complaints about shipping, quality, or service, trust your instincts and look elsewhere.

Authenticity and quality aren't mysterious. **Real products have signs:** packaging should never be cheap or poorly assembled. Spelling errors, blurry print, or mismatched logos can indicate counterfeits. Be wary of missing or unfamiliar manufacturer names that don't appear on trusted medical sites. Packaging should have tamper-evident seals; missing or broken seals are warning signs. The product itself should be consistent in color, texture, and smell every time. If you notice differences between bottles from the same brand, stop and reach out to customer support before using the product.

Understanding a COA

This is less daunting once you know what to look for. A legitimate COA lists the product's batch number, test date, and the independent lab performing the analysis. It should verify that the main ingredient matches what's on the label. Test results should show purity (usually as a percentage), presence of heavy metals (should read "ND" for not detected or show very low levels), microbial contamination, and, if relevant, solvent residues. It may also check for allergens like gluten or dairy. See Resources for a sample COA.

When reviewing COAs, start by matching the batch number on your product to the COA. If they don't match, press for answers or avoid the product. Check the lab's name; reputable labs have a clear online presence and often display their accreditations (like ISO 17025). Be skeptical of COAs that look plain, are missing letterheads, or appear like generic templates. Some sellers attempt to present fake or outdated analyses. If in doubt, contact the lab directly—reputable labs often handle such queries.

Independent laboratory verification is the gold standard. Some suppliers send samples to external labs with no financial interest in the product—exactly what you want. These independent labs use advanced tests like HPLC (high-performance liquid chromatography) or mass spectrometry to confirm ingredients and check for toxins. If a supplier mentions "third-party testing" but refuses to share lab reports or shows only internal data, that's insufficient. True independence means unbiased and legitimate results.

Supplier Due Diligence Checklist

Keep this checklist handy for purchasing:

- Are all product ingredients clearly listed?
- Is there a recent COA with batch number and lab contact information?
- Is the packaging professional and error-free?
- Does customer service respond to questions?
- Are there detailed, credible customer reviews?
- Is independent laboratory verification provided?
- Does the COA match your product's batch number?
- Is the lab named on the COA reputable and easily reached?
- Are purity and contaminant levels clearly within safe limits?
- Can you independently verify the manufacturer's reputation?

If you can answer "yes" to these, you're on firmer ground. Trust is built on transparency and evidence—not just hope or urgency.

Veterinary vs. Pharmaceutical-Grade Products

When you're weighing your options for sourcing repurposed drugs, the choice between veterinary and pharmaceutical-grade products gets real—fast. The two are not created equal, and the differences go far beyond the price tag or the picture of a dog or horse on the box. Pharmaceutical-grade products are manufactured for humans, following strict regulations that control every step from raw ingredients to finished tablets. Every batch must meet consistent standards for purity, potency, and absence of harmful byproducts. The fillers, dyes, and binders—called excipients—are chosen and tested for human safety, and there's a record of each step. Regulatory bodies like the FDA or EMA oversee pharmaceutical manufacturing, so you're far less likely to run into unknown surprises.

Veterinary products, on the other hand, are designed for animals with guidelines that aren't as strict as those for human medicines. The active ingredient—like fenbendazole or ivermectin—is usually the same molecule as in the pharmaceutical version, but what surrounds it can be a wild card. Veterinary pastes, granules, or chewables often have flavorings, artificial colors, or preservatives that are fine for a dog's belly but not ideal for a human dealing with cancer or a sensitive gut. Sometimes, the sweeteners or suspending agents are poorly tolerated, especially in large amounts or by people with allergies. Purity requirements are less rigid, so you might see more batch-to-batch variation. That said, some veterinary products are manufactured by the same companies making human medicines, just on different lines. It's all about knowing what you're really getting.

Purity standards and excipients are where things get interesting—and tricky. In pharmaceutical-grade drugs, the law requires strict testing not only for the main ingredient but also for everything else that's in the pill or liquid. Excipients like microcrystalline cellulose, magnesium stearate, or lactose are chosen for their safety in humans. For veterinary products, especially those made for large animals, excipients might include propylene glycol, artificial flavors, or food dyes. These additives can cause allergic reactions, stomach upset, or—rarely—other adverse effects in humans. The active ingredient may be present at the labeled dose, but the amount can sometimes swing a little higher or lower than you'd expect. Consistency from one package to the next is not guaranteed.

The risks and benefits of each option can't be ignored. Pharmaceutical-grade drugs are usually safer for people, with reliable dosing and fewer unknowns. The drawback is access—sometimes you need a prescription, or the cost is sky-high, or the drug isn't approved for your specific use. That's where veterinary products find their way into the conversation. They're often easier to buy online, come in larger packages, and cost much less. They offer an option when nothing else is available or affordable. But the risks include inconsistent dosage, possible contaminants, or excipients that don't play nicely with the human body. There's also the legal gray area—using animal drugs for people is off-label and not officially recommended, even though many desperate patients go this route.

Sometimes, using a veterinary product is acceptable—if you can't access the pharmaceutical-grade version, or you know exactly what's in the veterinary formula and you've checked for problematic excipients. For instance, some fenbendazole powders or tablets have only the active drug and a safe base like cornstarch. In those cases, people have reported using them with careful measurement and record-keeping. You should avoid products with a long list of artificial flavors, colors, or preservatives. If you have allergies, do a careful ingredient check before swallowing anything new. When in doubt, reach out to the manufacturer to request a full ingredient list.

Quality indicators can help tip you off to a safer product.

Look for consistent packaging with clear labeling—batch numbers, expiration dates, and company contact information should be present and readable. The powder or tablet should look and smell as expected: no strange colors, odd odors, or visible clumping. If you notice changes in color or texture between batches, set it aside until you can verify it's safe. Packaging that arrives sealed and intact is another good sign; anything with broken seals or loose powder in the box should make you pause. Also, some reputable vet brands have been in business for years and have a track record of quality—these are preferable if you can't get pharmaceutical-grade supplies.

You're not alone in feeling overwhelmed by all these details. Staying safe means asking about every ingredient, weighing risks versus benefits, and trusting your gut if something feels off. Document everything you use and how you respond to it. And when possible, seek out support groups or trusted healthcare professionals who can help you double-check your choices before moving forward.

Reputable Suppliers and Red Flags

Searching for a trustworthy place to buy repurposed drugs can feel overwhelming—everyone claims to offer miracle cures, but only a few are genuine. When so much is at stake, these decisions are nerve-wracking. Reputable online vendors share key qualities: their website clearly lists a physical address and phone number, and they offer responsive, live customer service. Transparent vendors readily answer questions about sourcing, ingredients, and quality controls; they don't dodge or give generic answers. Their sites are professional: clear product photos, accurate descriptions, and no wild health claims or gaudy banners.

Cancer drugs require extra vigilance. Be wary of websites overloaded with pop-ups, poor English, or endlessly shifting product names. Reliable suppliers rarely use aggressive sales tactics like urgent "limited stock!" alerts, unless demand genuinely exceeds supply. Avoid sites that insist on untraceable payments (Western Union, cryptocurrency) or ask for banking info in suspicious ways. If customer support only generates automated replies or remains silent, consider it a strong red flag. Always search for independent reviews—forums, Reddit, and cancer support groups often reveal honest experiences. If you can't find feedback or see repeated reports of missing or fake products, move on.

Counterfeit products

Counterfeit products aren't always easy to spot but learning to recognize their patterns is essential. Fake packaging often has spelling mistakes, fuzzy logos, or lacks manufacturer details. Pills that differ from official descriptions—wrong color, chipped, or with a strange smell—should not be trusted. Compare items to brand photos on manufacturer websites for accuracy. Watch for inconsistencies across orders, such as changes in tablet shape, size, or texture. Pills that are crumbly, moist, or overly powdery are often poor-quality fakes and should be discarded. Inferior production methods and questionable ingredients are common telltale signs.

When researching online, such as for manufacturers, it's important to make sure a website is the official one and not a counterfeit. Start by checking the web address (URL) carefully—official sites usually use the company or organization's exact name and end in trusted extensions like .com, .org, or a verified country domain. Look for small spelling changes or extra words, which are common signs of fake sites. Confirm the site has a secure connection (https:// and a padlock symbol). You can also cross-check the website link on trusted sources like the company's verified social media pages, government registries, or reputable directories. If prices, claims, or downloads seem too good to be true, proceed with caution. Taking a moment to verify these details can protect you from scams, malware, and misinformation.

Product-specific issues crop up frequently in patient groups. For fenbendazole, many turn to veterinary brands for affordability and availability, but this carries risks. Stick with brands known for consistency, like Panacur C, popular in animal clinics. Powders are easier to measure, but scrutinize ingredients—extra flavors, dyes, or additives can cause reactions. For ivermectin, human-grade tablets are safest; veterinary formulations (pastes, liquids) may contain animal additives unsuitable for humans. Always check labels and look for credible patient reviews. Some generics vary in quality between batches; if you doubt your product, contact the supplier for clarification or a replacement.

Other repurposed drugs like mebendazole and nitazoxanide are typically available as human pharmaceuticals, sometimes requiring a prescription by country. Avoid "grey market" pharmacies touting miracle cures or offering to ship worldwide without documentation—these are risky. The best approach is to consult patient support communities for up-to-date lists of reputable sources. Such groups often maintain vetted supplier lists based on collective user feedback.

Domestic versus international sourcing presents another challenge. Buying locally is preferable—there's less risk, quicker shipping, and stronger consumer protections. Domestic sellers answer to local agencies and are likelier to follow regulations. However, if drugs are unavailable due to prescription restrictions or shortages, some turn to international vendors, which are harder to vet and present additional risks like customs delays or legal gray areas. Imported shipments might be seized or lost, so know your country's rules and keep all receipts, correspondence, and packaging in case you need to demonstrate what you ordered.

It may seem daunting, but careful research and diligence in choosing suppliers helps you avoid dangerous scams and unsafe products. Every extra check is a layer of protection for your health.

Storage, Handling, and Shelf Life

Once you acquire your medications—be it fenbendazole, ivermectin, or another agent—the crucial next step is keeping them safe and effective. Improper storage can quickly ruin a product: a single mishap, like leaving medicine in a hot car or a damp bathroom, can render a drug useless or even unsafe.

Choose a cool, dry place away from sunlight to store your medications. A kitchen cabinet far from the stove, or a bedroom dresser drawer, is better than a humid bathroom. Always follow manufacturer instructions—if the label mentions refrigeration, avoiding light, or another requirement, take it seriously. Heat and sunlight degrade many drugs, while moisture can cause tablets to crumble, powders to clump, or capsules to stick. A solution can be as simple as using a plastic container with a tight lid, clearly labeled with the drug name, dose, and opening date, and keeping it away from windows and heat sources. This extra step beats discovering your medicine has degraded or spoiled.

Inspect your medications each time you use them. Are colors off? Do powders look clumpy or musty? Any odd smells or visible changes can mean a product is no longer safe or effective. Even subtle shifts can spell trouble. Don't take risks: discard anything that looks, smells, or feels wrong; at the very least, contact the manufacturer and discuss it with them.

Expiration dates matter, too. These are based on tested stability, guiding you on when the medication should still perform as intended. Using drugs past this date risks reduced potency or, occasionally, harmful byproducts. Mark expiration dates prominently on every bottle or packet. If you break large packages down, transfer the original expiration date and batch number to each new container. This simplifies rotation and minimizes waste.

Potency can decline before expiration if storage advice isn't followed. Weekly pill organizers, for example, must be airtight and shielded from light and heat. Don't mix old and new batches in the same container; finish the older supply first. If in doubt about a product's integrity, contact your supplier or manufacturer—many will advise or even test samples if you have batch info and purchase details.

Handling safely extends beyond storage. Wash hands both before and after handling medications. Always use a clean, dry tool for measuring powders—never your fingers. Clean up spills immediately, and keep all medications out of reach of children and pets. For liquid forms, use the provided measuring tool or a pharmacy syringe; household spoons aren't accurate. Use a pill splitter for tablets, not a knife, for more reliable dosing. Dispose of expired or unused medications via pharmacy take-back programs, not in the trash or toilet (unless the label specifically says so).

If you're taking multiple agents or supplements, keep a medication log with storage details, opening dates, and any changes you notice. This helps you catch issues early. Store each agent in its own clearly marked container. If you have trouble managing this yourself, consider enlisting a family member for weekly organizing.

Amid the stress of illness, these habits can feel like extra work, but routine makes them easy and automatic. The payoff is peace of mind, fewer wasted medications, and reassurance that every dose you take retains its full effectiveness.

In summary, proper storage and handling aren't just about protecting a product; they're an investment in your safety. A little planning reduces waste and accidental exposures, and ensures each dose supports your treatment. The next chapter will guide you in weaving these principles into a protocol that fits your daily life.

Chapter 8
Integrative Oncology — Bridging Standard and Alternative Approaches

Defining Integrative Oncology

You've probably heard the term "integrative oncology" and wondered what it means in practice, especially when faced with overwhelming treatment choices. You might wish someone could simply connect all the dots for you. That's what integrative oncology does—it's not about picking between conventional medicine and alternative therapies, but about blending both to fit each individual. It combines standard treatments like chemotherapy or surgery with evidence-based adjuncts such as dietary changes, stress management, or non-toxic drugs. The philosophy is treating you as a whole person—respecting your values, preferences, and needs, not just your diagnosis.

In practical terms, integrative oncology offers you real choices. You're not trapped on a single path. If you want to pair your oncologist's chemo protocol with a ketogenic diet, meditation, or supplements with supporting evidence, you can. Curious about hyperbaric oxygen or repurposed drugs like fenbendazole, but want to stay with standard care? That's possible too. The key is a both-and approach instead of either-or. You become an active part of the conversation, encouraged to ask questions and share preferences, rather than just following orders.

At its heart, integrative oncology puts you—the patient—first. In conventional medicine, it's easy to feel reduced to a case file. Integrative oncology reverses that. You're encouraged to express what matters, whether it's managing pain without extra meds, keeping your mind clear for family, or having energy for a daily walk. Your care team listens not in medical jargon, but with respect for your goals and concerns. If you propose something new or different, it's considered thoughtfully, not dismissed outright.

The beauty of this approach is the careful blending of conventional treatments with evidence-backed adjuncts: acupuncture for nausea, yoga for anxiety, or dietary changes to enhance your metabolism. Integrative oncology isn't about chasing every "miracle cure" from the internet. It's about sifting fact from hype, working with professionals who stay current on both mainstream and holistic research. The therapies suggested have actual evidence behind them—scientific studies, case reports, or long-established traditional use—and you're encouraged to ask for and review the proof yourself.

The Personalized Medicine Clinic is an example of integrative medicine that is focused on cancer and metabolic therapies: https://www.personalizedmedicinemd.co/

Safety remains the foundation. With so many therapies available—some effective, some potentially risky—it's natural to feel unsure. This is why clear communication is vital: always tell your providers about every supplement, protocol, or symptom. Your team needs a complete picture to watch for possible interactions and red flags. Good integrative oncology teams welcome this openness. If your questions or interests in alternatives are met with judgment, it's a signal to find a more receptive provider.

Personal preference is more important than many realize. You're not just along for the ride—you help decide the course and to steer. Some will want to pursue every option; others may value comfort and quality of life over aggressive treatment. Integrative oncology respects and supports your decisions without guilt or pressure. If guided imagery helps you relax during infusions, or switching to organic foods restores a sense of control, those are valid and personal choices for you alone to make.

Interactive Reflection:

What Matters Most to You? Pause now, grab a notebook or notes app, and jot down answers to these:

- What are your three top health priorities?
- Are there side effects or symptoms you most want to avoid?
- What beliefs and values drive your treatment choices?
- What does a "good day" mean for you at this stage? Check this list before major decisions or appointments. Bring it along to keep conversations focused on what truly matters to you.

Integrative oncology blends science with empathy, offers you choices with safety, and always respects the whole person, not just the diagnosis.

Real-World Synergy Examples

A lot of people ask me, "Can I actually combine things like metabolic diets or repurposed meds with chemo or radiation?" I see this all the time—people feeling stuck between two worlds, not knowing if it's possible to bridge them safely. But you can, and many have. The synergy between conventional and alternative therapies is not a fantasy. It's real, and it's happening right now in the lives of patients who refuse to give up after the first round of side effects or discouraging news. Take ketogenic diets, for example. Some folks who were exhausted from chemo, barely able to keep food down, find that switching to a low-carb, high-fat plan gave them a steadier kind of energy. They stopped having wild sugar swings. Their nausea eased. They had improvement in overall health, even during treatment. Some research suggests a ketogenic diet can make cancer cells more sensitive to chemo and radiation, helping treatments work better. It's not universal, and not every doctor is on board, but for those who try it, the difference can be remarkable.

Sometimes the most powerful synergy comes from outside the pharmacy or kitchen. It's in the stories of people who used **acupuncture or guided imagery to manage pain, or who turned to yoga or breathwork for anxiety** while still attending every medical appointment. One man with lymphatic cancer said that meditation and breathwork were what made him able to keep showing up for radiation—not because it cured him, but because it made the process bearable. He slept better, panicked less, and felt more like himself.

What ties all these examples together isn't just the therapies—it's the willingness to experiment, document, and keep communication lines open. No one approach works for everyone, but when people combine what modern medicine offers with evidence-based alternatives, they often find more hope and fewer side effects. If you're considering a combined path, keep records, ask questions, and don't be afraid to take your findings to your next appointment. This space—where mainstream and alternative meet—is where some of the most meaningful progress happens for real people like you.

Working with Healthcare Teams

Building your cancer care team can feel overwhelming. Juggling oncologists, nutritionists, and naturopaths—each with different perspectives—can be difficult. Yet, with cancer, no single provider has all the answers. You deserve a team that respects your choices, discusses risks and benefits, and sees you as more than a protocol. Conventional primary care doctors and oncologists are stuck on the "Standard of Care" hamster wheel, and not permitted to suggest alternatives. Wanting more than the standard treatment makes you proactive, not "difficult." It's your body and your life.

Clear communication with your care team is crucial. When exploring adjunct therapies—such as fenbendazole, IV vitamin C, or a metabolic diet—document everything: treatments, dosages, dates, side effects, and symptoms. Use a notebook or app to log these details and take them to every appointment. This ongoing record helps both you and your providers spot patterns—improvements or early side effects. You don't need medical jargon, just honest, dated notes. This approach shows you're an engaged participant and gives your team specifics to respond to, not just impressions.

Discussing alternatives with doctors can trigger anxiety, especially when you fear dismissal. An honest, curious approach—rather than confrontation—is often best. Say, for instance: "I've been researching adjunct therapies that others use with conventional treatment. I'd like your input on safety or possible interactions." When adding something new, ask: "Can we review the evidence together? I value your expertise but want to advocate for myself." If faced with skepticism, calmly explain your motivations: "My goal is to improve quality of life and resilience during treatment. I'm not rejecting your care; I'd like to complement it." When resistance persists, rely on the facts: "I keep detailed records and want your input if you see concerns." Even if you aren't met with enthusiasm, keeping dialogue open gradually builds mutual respect. And this doesn't just benefit you. An open-minded practitioner can may actually learn useful tidbits from you and your data.

Assembling your integrative care team takes effort. Start by asking current providers if they know integrative oncologists, NDs, or nutritionists experienced in cancer care. Seek those who listen more than lecture and openly discuss dietary interventions, repurposed drugs, or complementary therapies. Quality team members will weigh pros and cons based on evidence. Vet new providers by noting how they answer tough questions: Do they admit what they don't know? Are they willing to collaborate? Can they share references or case studies from their practice?

Coordination often breaks down—providers might not communicate with each other. Share your medication and supplement list with every provider. Ask them to share labs and notes, and try to arrange joint calls or group emails. Be fully transparent about all interventions, even if you fear judgment—the risk of hidden interactions grows with multiple therapies. If you have an advocate—a family member, friend, or patient navigator—enlist their help tracking appointments, organizing records, and pushing for team communication. Especially when you're tired or overwhelmed, an advocate can remind you of your priorities, ensure your questions are heard, and prevent things from slipping through the cracks.

Patient navigators and advocates

Many hospital systems offer invaluable navigation services at no cost. Navigators understand medical red tape, explain jargon, arrange second opinions, and help with referrals. A good navigator respects your preferences and helps build a supportive, individualized team. They can also catch insurance issues, since coverage sometimes depends on how things are documented. Don't hesitate to seek a navigator—or to meet with several until you find someone supportive.

Ultimately, you're not seeking perfect agreement among your providers. Your goal is a group that respects your voice, keeps an open mind, and supports your vision of healing—even if it means learning together along the way.

Sample Scripts for Talking to Doctors

Discussing alternative protocols with your doctor can be daunting; you may be concerned that you'd come across like someone who believes everything he/she reads read online. If your doctor is open-minded, start with honesty and humility: "I've read about adjunct therapies some people with cancer use. I want to be safe and possibly find something to complement, not interfere with, my treatment. Can we look at this together?" Doctors who value partnership will appreciate your transparency. They might not know every protocol, but most will look at research or listen to your reasoning. If they're curious, bring brief, relevant articles or handouts. Sometimes, this leads to wider discussions—such as clinical trials or safe supplement use—that might not have come up otherwise.

However, not every provider welcomes alternative topics. Some see "alternative" as "potentially dangerous." If you sense skepticism, reframe your approach. Instead of asking for permission, say: "I'm considering this protocol because I read about its use in cancer. I'd like your help to spot any safety issues or possible drug interactions." This shows you're being proactive, not reckless. If skepticism persists, calmly add, "I value your expertise and won't stop any treatment you recommend. I just want the best chance possible." If the conversation grows tense or dismissive, remember that seeking a second opinion is valid. Another provider may offer the openness or experience you need.

When facing outright refusals or dismissals—perhaps hearing, "There's no evidence for that," or "I can't be involved if you do this"—stay composed. You might reply, "I hear your concerns and know you want what's best for me. I want to try this because it gives me hope and a sense of control. I'll continue all prescribed treatments and will alert you to any changes or side effects." If your choices are refused outright, document the conversation and consider finding support elsewhere—an integrative oncologist, naturopathic doctor, or other care team member. Your health is worth finding the right fit.

Clear records of every protocol, supplement, and conversation are essential—a real safety net. After appointments, record what was discussed, the doctor's response, and follow-up recommendations. This running log helps when doctors change or when recalling conversations from stressful visits. It also makes communicating across multiple providers easier—keeping everyone informed and preventing details from getting lost.

Having written records can also help defend your choices with insurance, new providers, or concerned family members. You don't need a special app—just something consistent you'll actually use.

Ultimately, these conversations are about mutual respect—for yourself and your care team. The goal isn't to win arguments or prove someone wrong, but to build trust, protect your safety, and ensure your choices are well-informed and supported. You deserve a team that listens, even if they're unsure, and a space where you can share hopes, fears, and plans without being dismissed.

Sometimes these talks will be smooth; other times, awkward or disappointing. Remember: you're the one living through this. You have every right to ask questions, explore options, and insist on respect. These skills will serve you in every major decision, not just in cancer care.

Blending openness with diligent record-keeping empowers you to track your progress and decisions. As you continue to develop your plan, the next step is designing a truly personalized protocol—one that respects both your biology and values, helping you regain a sense of control.

Chapter 9
Safety, Monitoring, and Legal Considerations

Side Effects, Contraindications, and Drug Interactions

Standing in your kitchen with a new medication brings anxiety and hope, especially when uncertainty about safety lingers. Knowing the risks and warning signs of these therapies before you begin is essential.

Fenbendazole, though famously gentle in dogs, isn't risk-free for humans. Most users experience mild effects—stomach upset, loose stools, or brief headaches. Occasionally, people report a rash or lingering fatigue. Mebendazole, closely related, causes similar side effects but can also lower white blood cells or irritate the liver, especially at high doses or with long use, so regular liver function tests are recommended—particularly if you're adding other liver-stressing medications. Nitazoxanide may cause nausea, cramps, or oddly colored urine (harmless but startling). Ivermectin, safely used for millions, sometimes causes dizziness, itching, or swelling; rarely, it leads to blurred vision or confusion, which signal it's time to stop and get checked.

Certain people should avoid these drugs. Fenbendazole and mebendazole aren't suitable for those with severe liver disease, blood disorders, or known allergies to benzimidazoles. Nitazoxanide should be avoided by those with chronic liver or severe kidney conditions. Ivermectin is unsafe for those allergic to it or with a history of neurologic conditions such as seizures. Pregnant or breastfeeding women should be especially cautious, as safety is unproven for developing babies.

Drug interactions are a concern, especially with cancer medications. Many chemotherapy and targeted therapies use the CYP450 liver enzyme, the same pathway for ivermectin, mebendazole, and most drugs used by clinicians. Combining these raises drug levels and toxicity risks—such as jaundice, confusion, mouth sores, and ongoing vomiting. Risks of low blood counts, liver injury, and nerve problems increase when stacking these or multiple repurposed drugs without regular monitoring.

Red Flag Symptom Checklist

- Severe abdominal pain
- Dark urine or yellowing of skin/eyes
- Unexplained bruising or bleeding
- High fever or chills
- Sudden vision changes
- Intense headache with neck stiffness
- Confusion, slurred speech, or new weakness

If any of these occur, stop all non-essential medications and contact your doctor or urgent care. Refer to your notes for what you've taken and when, to help your care team respond quickly.

Combining Repurposed Drugs with Chemotherapy or Immunotherapy

If you're considering mixing repurposed drugs with chemo or immunotherapy, you're not alone. Safe integration isn't about taking everything at once; it involves careful layering, timing, and open communication with your medical team. It's best to introduce new agents gradually—typically starting one repurposed drug a week or two before your next chemo cycle—while monitoring for unusual symptoms or lab results. If all stays stable, you may be able to continue the repurposed drug during treatment, though some people choose to pause it during the toughest chemo days to avoid extra strain on the liver or immune system.

Some protocols advise stopping drugs like fenbendazole or ivermectin two days before chemo and restarting three days after, allowing your body time to recover. Others follow a "concurrent" approach, using both at lower daily doses with careful hydration and monitoring. There's no universal plan, but gradual introductions and staggered starts are generally safest. **Visual schedules—color-coded calendars marking chemo, repurposed meds, and rest days—can help you track doses and lower anxiety.**

Monitoring is essential. Get labs (liver enzymes, kidney function, white blood counts) weekly or biweekly to catch issues early.

Many medications — including a large number of chemotherapy and targeted cancer drugs — are processed by the liver using specific enzyme pathways. Two of the most common are called CYP3A4 and CYP2C19. These enzymes act like traffic controllers, helping the body break drugs down at the right speed so they are effective but not harmful. When more than one medication or supplement uses the same pathway, they can compete with or interfere with each other.

This doesn't mean combinations are unsafe or should be avoided. It means they should be cross-checked intentionally. Some substances slow these enzymes down, which can cause a drug to stay in the body longer and increase side effects. Others speed the enzymes up, which can cause a drug to clear too quickly and reduce its effectiveness. This is especially relevant when combining chemotherapy with repurposed drugs, antibiotics, or certain supplements. Taking a moment to check for known interactions — or to discuss timing, dosing, or monitoring with your care team — helps ensure each part of your plan is working with your body, not against it.

Real-world experiences offer hope and reminders for caution. Some have seen tumors shrink and side effects ease, but others ran into trouble by stacking too many agents too quickly, leading to severe side effects or ER visits. These stories highlight the importance of restraint, close tracking, and steady communication.

Monitoring for Success: Biomarkers, Imaging, and Symptom Tracking

When you start any new protocol, especially something outside the mainstream, you want solid proof that what you're doing is really working. Guesswork is stressful. You deal with enough uncertainty already. That's why I believe in tracking everything you can—objectively and subjectively—to help guide your decisions and give you confidence in the steps you're taking. One of the most reliable ways to judge progress is through cancer biomarkers—measured in your blood or other bodily fluids. These aren't just numbers; they often reflect how aggressive or quiet the cancer is behaving. Markers like PSA for prostate, CEA for colon, CA-125 for ovarian, or even newer ones like ctDNA (circulating tumor cells DNA) are more than acronyms—they're early warning systems, and sometimes they reveal improvement long before you feel better or before a scan changes. Imaging—CT, PET, MRI, or ultrasound—shows the physical story: are tumors shrinking, stable, or growing? Comparing these images over time, side by side, can clarify trends that might otherwise get lost in the noise of daily ups and downs.

But numbers and pictures only tell part of the story. How you actually feel, day in and day out, matters just as much. This is where your daily log shines—not just of side effects, but of energy levels, appetite, sleep, pain, mood, and anything else that changes. Use a notebook or a phone app. The act of writing things down helps you notice subtle shifts, both good and bad. It also arms you with facts when talking to your care team. Maybe you realize your fatigue spikes after starting a new supplement, or that nausea eases when you change your dose timing.

You might find it helpful to use templates for recording each scan or lab result. Take these to appointments, email them to your provider, or share them with your support group. Sharing this tracking data helps your doctors see what's really happening between visits and lets them spot red flags—or successes—faster than relying on memory alone. These records don't just empower you; they make your whole team stronger.

When to Adjust or Discontinue a Protocol

There's nothing more unsettling than realizing the plan you've put your faith in might need to change. Sometimes, you get a gut feeling—maybe your energy drops, your appetite disappears, or you just don't feel right. Other times, it's more concrete: lab results slip out of range, or your scans show something you didn't expect. When these moments happen, it's easy to panic or feel stuck. The truth is, making changes is part of the process. Knowing when to adjust or stop a protocol is a kind of wisdom that comes from listening to your body, paying attention to the data, and being honest about what's working and what's not.

Red flags aren't always dramatic, but they do demand respect. If you notice steady weight loss you can't explain, weakness, swelling in your legs, new or worsening pain, or problems like confusion or persistent vomiting, that's your cue to slow down and reassess. Sometimes the signs are subtle—like growing fatigue, brain fog, or a mood shift. When you view the process as fluid, you can look at these, these not as failures, but as signals to pause and ask: Is this protocol helping, or is it time to tweak something? If the answer isn't clear, step back and review your logs: What changed right before these symptoms appeared? Did you add a new supplement, increase a dose, or stack two therapies together? Has anything in your life changed—diet, stress, hydration? Are you taking something at a different time of day? Did you skip meals or lose sleep?

Troubleshooting comes down to stripping things back and moving one step at a time. If you're on more than one agent, cut back to the basics—keep only what you're sure is safe, then reintroduce others slowly if symptoms settle. This process can feel tedious, but it beats shooting in the dark. Sometimes, it means stopping everything for a few days and letting your system reset.

You never have to do this alone. Reach out to your medical team when things get murky—the nurse, oncologist, or even a trusted pharmacist can help sort out what's urgent and what can wait. And I know I keep saying this, but it helps to take concrete notes—dates, symptoms, and any changes you've made—so you can review together with your care team. If your provider suggests stopping or adjusting a drug, ask for their reasoning and write it down. Don't be afraid to get a second opinion if something doesn't sit right. This collaborative approach not only keeps you safer but reminds you that your voice matters in every decision.

Off-Label Legal Landscape

When I first started looking into fenbendazole and ivermectin, I realized just how much confusion and fear swirl around the words "off-label," "not FDA-approved," and "veterinary use." In the U.S., "off-label" simply means using a drug in a way not specifically listed on its label, but prescribed by a physician. This practice is common—even standard cancer drugs are often used off-label for types or stages not officially listed in their paperwork. What throws people off is when a medicine isn't FDA-approved for any human use, like fenbendazole, which is purely a veterinary product. You can buy it at pet stores or online, but technically, it's not made for people. Doctors can't prescribe it, and pharmacists won't fill a script for it. Using it is legal for animals, but if you take it yourself, you step into a gray zone; the law isn't clear-cut, but it's generally not a criminal act unless you're selling or making false claims.

Rules change by country. In the UK, off-label prescriptions are allowed if a doctor believes it's in your best interest, but veterinary drugs for humans are a no-go. Canada follows similar lines: off-label is fine with a doctor's supervision, but importing or using animal meds for yourself is technically prohibited. Australia is strictest—customs can seize unapproved drugs, and heavy fines exist. Across the EU, each country has its own quirks, but the pattern is clear: off-label is sometimes tolerated, but self-medicating with animal drugs is discouraged and may break regulations. In the U.S., some people use personal importation loopholes for a three-month supply, but this is always at your own risk. If you're unsure, consult a lawyer familiar with health law or reach out to patient advocacy groups that specialize in alternative medicine rights. Clear records and honesty go a long way in protecting yourself if questions ever arise.

Ordering unapproved or veterinary drugs online carries real risks. Packages can be seized by customs, leaving you out of money or even facing legal scrutiny. You might get counterfeit or contaminated products. To lower your risk, research suppliers carefully, avoid large orders, and never claim a package contains "medicine" if questioned by customs. If you're working with a medical team, be transparent about everything you use. Keep all receipts, batch numbers, and correspondence.

Veterinary Drug Use Patient Rights and Myths

Many standard therapies actually started as off-label before gaining full approval. In alternative medicine, off-label may include using drugs like fenbendazole or mebendazole (designed for parasites in animals) for other uses, even when evidence is early or anecdotal. Such flexibility can be both a lifeline and a challenge, as it requires you and your care team to carefully weigh risks and benefits.

There are several myths about off-label and veterinary drug use. Some believe it's illegal, but doctors in most countries can prescribe human drugs off-label if it's in your best interest. Another myth is that only desperate or uninformed patients pursue off-label treatments. In fact, many well-informed people opt for these after research and discussions with their doctors. Some fear doctors will drop them as patients for asking about off-label options. While some providers may hesitate, you are always entitled to ask questions, raise possibilities, and make informed choices. It is your doctor's responsibility to advise and facilitate; it is your responsibility to yourself to make informed decisions.

Your patient rights are stronger than you might expect. You can request all your records, seek second opinions, and bring outside research or protocols to your doctor's attention. You have the right to refuse treatment or suggest alternatives, even if your doctor disagrees. If you want to explore veterinary drugs, be honest about your intentions and ask your doctor to help monitor labs and symptoms. This isn't just about autonomy—it's about safety and shared responsibility.

Good documentation is vital for both ethical and practical reasons. Keep a simple log of doses, symptoms, questions, and your care team's advice. This record helps protect you and keeps your care team informed. Responsible off-label use is about transparency, teamwork, and ensuring your right to participate in every aspect of your care—not secrecy or recklessness.

Insurance, Documentation, and Protecting Treatment Choices

Dealing with insurance while exploring alternative treatments can feel like wrestling a shadow. If you've ever sat on hold for an hour only to be told a treatment isn't covered, you know the frustration all too well. When you step outside the narrow lanes of standard care—adding a repurposed drug, trying metabolic therapies, or seeking integrative support—insurance companies often draw a hard line. In many plans, coverage for non-standard or "experimental" therapies is excluded, and repurposed meds like fenbendazole or even more mainstream approaches like hyperbaric oxygen therapy may not make the cut. Some plans will deny claims for anything not FDA-approved for your diagnosis, regardless of evidence or medical need. That means you might pay out-of-pocket, or you could find yourself needing to fight back against a denial.

The backbone of any appeal or dispute is documentation. I can't stress this enough: write down everything. Keep every test result, doctor's note, prescription, receipt, and email about your care—whether it's standard or alternative. If your doctor supports your protocol, ask them to write a letter explaining the medical necessity, even if it's off-label or not yet mainstream. Record the dates of every call with your insurer, and get the names of representatives. Save denial letters, as well as your responses. If you appeal a decision, include scientific articles or case studies that back your request. Sometimes, persistence and a thick folder of evidence can turn a "no" into a "yes," or at least get you partial reimbursement.

If you get a denial, don't lose hope. Most policies have a formal appeals process—usually two or three steps. Submit everything in writing and keep copies. You can also ask your provider to resubmit the claim with more specific language. If that fails, contact your state's insurance commissioner or ombudsman. Occasionally, advocacy organizations will help patients with appeals, especially for high-cost or life-saving treatments.

Sometimes, the fight takes a legal turn. If you believe your insurer or provider is discriminating against you for seeking alternatives, legal aid groups or cancer advocacy organizations might step in. You may have rights under state or federal law to pursue treatments or appeal unfair denials. Don't be afraid to ask for help. Support groups and online communities can offer tips and sample letters.

Wrapping up this chapter, remember that protecting your treatment choices means staying organized, documenting every step, and calling on help when you need it. Insurance hurdles can be daunting, but with good records and support, you can push back. In the next chapter, we'll dig into building a protocol that fits your unique story and health goals.

Chapter 10
Creating Your Personalized Protocol

Mapping Your Journey: Flowcharts and Decision Trees

Building a personalized cancer care protocol often feels like piecing together a confusing puzzle, especially given the array of options and uncertainties. During my research journey it became clear that most people never discover all their options, and those that do never see them visually laid out—even though such visuals can help bring order to chaos. That’s where flowcharts and decision trees come in. These tools aren’t reserved for professionals; they're essential for anyone wanting to clearly see their choices and regain some control.

Visual decision tools quickly dispel confusion. Seeing options mapped—yes/no, if this/then that—is like shining a light in a dark room. You don't have to remember every detail; the chart does that for you, laying out steps logically. This visual support is crucial when emotions or fatigue make complex decisions even harder. A flowchart acts as an anchor, making it easier to focus on what matters with each decision point.

Here's how these tools work in practice: A flowchart starting with, "What type of cancer am I facing?" The path splits into options like breast, lung, or colon cancer, blood disorders, or rare tumors. Next, it considers your current treatment: chemotherapy, radiation, immunotherapy, or none. Maybe you're newly diagnosed, or maybe you've tried various protocols already. Each response leads to unique paths. If you're receiving treatment, the chart might prompt, "Is your doctor open to integrative therapies?" Each answer leads toward protocols safe to use in your situation.

At every stage, flowcharts clarify your key priorities. Are you aiming for remission, slowing disease progression, or simply improving quality of life? Your answer shapes the chart's next steps. If you prioritize shrinking a tumor pre-surgery, the flowchart may suggest combining metabolic therapies with repurposed drugs shown to help your cancer type. If your goal is symptom control during palliative care, it steers you toward supportive adjuncts and mind-body therapies.

The beauty of these tools is their adaptability. Cancer isn't static; your plan shouldn't be either. New life changes, side effects, or labs can shift your course quickly. Flowcharts and decision trees are meant to be revisited—print, mark up, and revise as things evolve. After months on a protocol, for example, check: Did side effects occur? Did lab markers improve? Just update your chart. This approach lets you stay proactive about your care rather than simply reacting to changes.

I've included a **decision tree protocol mapping tool** at the end of this chapter.

Interactive Element: Protocol Mapping Exercise

Take a quiet moment with the chart at the end of this chapter (or download it). It begins with your cancer type, then progresses to current treatment, and unfolds based on your answers. It discusses contraindications, and possible treatment categories to discuss with your oncologist. As specific decisions come up—like starting a new supplement or switching diets—follow the arrows to your next practical step. Keep this chart nearby so you can update it after each important change or discussion, or print a new one to complete.

Having your own protocol map is not just an exercise in organization—it's a way of reclaiming agency during an overwhelming process. Whether your path is straightforward or winding, this tangible guide makes each decision less intimidating and lets you communicate your choices clearly with your support team.

Creating Your Supplement Stack: What to Include and Why

Building a supplement stack is like assembling a targeted toolkit—every supplement should play a clear role and work well with others. "Stacking" means combining supplements that address different needs, such as inflammation, mitochondrial support, immunity, or detoxification. The goal is not to create a lengthy list, but to be strategic; your stack should reflect your personal goals, cancer type, and current treatments. Adding too many supplements at once can complicate things and make it difficult to tell what's actually effective or causing side effects.

A smart stack usually begins with supplements supported by credible evidence. Curcumin, found in turmeric, is popular for its anti-inflammatory effects and some anti-tumor evidence. Green tea extract (EGCG) is another frequent choice for its antioxidant properties and potential to slow tumor growth in lab studies. Medicinal mushrooms like turkey tail and reishi are recognized in integrative oncology for boosting immune function and possibly aiding recovery after chemotherapy. Omega-3 fatty acids (from fish oil) are valued for reducing chronic inflammation and supporting heart and brain health, which can suffer during cancer treatments. Vitamin D3 is essential since many people with cancer are deficient, and better levels are linked to improved outcomes and mood. Magnesium is widely used for sleep, muscle cramps, and stress. Melatonin, beyond aiding sleep, may also support immunity and have anti-cancer effects.

It's easy to get carried away and want to try every supplement you read about, but keeping your stack focused is important. Include only supplements with solid evidence or proven value in cancer care. Be cautious with trendy or minimally researched options like high-dose vitamin C or obscure herbal extracts. Stacking too many antioxidants, for example, can sometimes interfere with treatments such as radiation or certain chemotherapies. Additionally, some popular supplements—like St. John's wort or grapefruit extract—may dangerously interact with cancer drugs by affecting how your liver handles medications. Always check for potential interactions using a reliable drug interaction checker or consult a pharmacist familiar with integrative medicine.

Quality control is crucial. Purchase only supplements from reputable brands with batch numbers, expiration dates, and third-party lab testing for purity and contaminants. Pay special attention to details: for medicinal mushrooms, opt for products containing the fruiting body rather than just mycelium grown on grain; for fish oil, ensure it is independently tested for heavy metals. Avoid cheap knockoffs, especially from questionable online sources. Getting EPA (eicosapentaenoic acid) and DHA (docosahexaenoic acid), two main types of omega-3 fatty acids from food is superior to fish oil supplements that have often been found to be rancid. You can get adequate amounts from fish like salmon, herring, mackerel, and sardines, and pastured eggs. If you opt for a supplement, dosing accuracy is also key—start with the lowest recommended dose, and increase slowly while monitoring for side effects. Overdosing, especially on fat-soluble vitamins like D or A, can be harmful. Use pill organizers or reminders to avoid missing or doubling doses.

Your ideal stack will depend on your unique situation. During chemotherapy, the focus might shift toward immune support (medicinal mushrooms, vitamin D), gut health (probiotics), and managing stress (magnesium, melatonin). If following metabolic therapies like keto (which is strongly recommended, regardless of cancer type), electrolyte supplements—magnesium, sodium, potassium—can help prevent cramping and fatigue. For chronic inflammation, curcumin/turmeric, fish oil, and boswellia are popular. Those aiming for tumor suppression may combine curcumin, green tea extract, and melatonin, adding vitamin D if needed. It's essential to keep your medical team informed about all supplements you're taking. Provide a written list, including dosages and brands, to help prevent dangerous interactions or missed opportunities for support.

Build your supplement stack gradually and carefully. Track what you take, your reasons for adding it, and any changes you notice—positive or negative. This helps pinpoint what's effective and what isn't. Supplements should never replace a healthy diet or standard medical care, but when thoughtfully selected, they can improve your wellbeing and help your body better navigate the challenges of cancer and its treatment.

Avoiding Common Mistakes

When you're building your own protocol, it's easy to stumble into mistakes that can set you back or leave you second-guessing, and feels like learning a new language under pressure. Dosing errors is a common occurrence. Maybe you misread a label or get confused by milligrams versus grams, or lose track of whether it's time for your next dose. Even seasoned caregivers make mistakes here, especially when medications or supplements must be cycled on and off. Skipping days, doubling up after a missed dose, or stacking different agents without tracking—these can all mess with your progress or spark side effects. The best protection is having a set routine. Use tracking sheets, alarms, calendars, and a pillbox labeled for each day. Consistency in timing and dose helps your body adjust and makes it easier to notice what's helping and what's not.

Communication breakdowns with your care team can happen for endless reasons. You might feel nervous about bringing up alternative treatments, or fear being dismissed. Sometimes it's just that appointments are rushed or your oncologist seems too busy. But letting things slide or keeping your protocol secret can backfire. Not telling your doctor about new supplements or drugs can lead to dangerous interactions or missed warning signs. Honest, clear updates—written lists, logs of what you're taking, having your questions ready—make it easier for your care team to support you. Even if your provider isn't fully on board with every part of your plan, most want to keep you safe and will appreciate being kept in the loop. If you feel ignored or dismissed, it's worth seeking out a second opinion or a more open-minded practitioner. Your safety and progress matter far more than anyone's ego.

To make things easier, here's a checklist that can help bulletproof your protocol against common mistakes:

- Write down every medication, supplement, and dose on a single sheet—update this whenever you change anything.
- Set alarms for each dose using your phone or a clock that you see daily.
- Use a medication organizer with labeled compartments for each day and time slot.
- Before you order anything online, ask for a certificate of analysis and check the brand with a quick search for independent reviews. If you're unsure about a supplier, reach out to a support group or advocacy organization for recommendations.
- Always store everything in its original packaging with batch and expiration info visible. At every medical visit, bring your updated supplement/medication list and ask directly about possible interactions.
- If you start feeling new side effects, pause and review recent changes—sometimes less is more.
- And finally, remember to forgive yourself if you slip up. Cancer care is tough enough without beating yourself up over honest mistakes. You're learning, adapting, and doing your best—don't let fear of messing up stop you from moving forward.

Customizing by Cancer Type, Stage, and Treatment History

Personalizing your protocol means taking the science and shaping it to fit your own life. Even though the root problem is dysfunctional metabolism, as Dr. Thomas Seyfried has proven (hence the importance of a ketogenic diet), each tumor grows in its own environment, reacts to therapies in its own rhythm, and causes its own set of symptoms. The type, where it started, how far it's spread, and the treatments you've had before all matter. You need to see both the broad patterns and the fine details.

For example, someone with early-stage breast cancer who just had surgery faces different challenges from a person with advanced lung cancer who's already been through multiple lines of chemotherapy. In early stages, you might focus on strengthening your body between treatments, targeting any leftover cancer cells, and reducing risk of recurrence. Here, a protocol could lean more on metabolic therapies—like a tightly tracked ketogenic diet—and gentle repurposed drugs, since your immune system and organs are still relatively strong. If you're healing after surgery or prepping for radiation, you might add supplements known for tissue repair and inflammation control. Regular bloodwork and scans help track if your approach is working, and you can afford to make gradual adjustments.

On the other hand, with advanced or metastatic cancer, priorities often shift. Energy preservation, symptom control, and balancing side effects take the front seat. Tumors that have spread may have already adapted to outsmart standard treatments. In these cases, combining metabolic therapy (which is always the first line of defense) with carefully chosen repurposed drugs—like fenbendazole or ivermectin—can sometimes slow progression or ease symptoms, but you have to be careful. Here, stacking too many new therapies can overwhelm a body already taxed by years of treatment. You might need lower doses, longer rest periods, or extra liver and kidney monitoring. Sometimes it's not about aggressive tumor kill, but about keeping quality of life as high as possible and gently nudging the disease into a slower pattern. You may also need to weigh new risks: for example, if your bone marrow is weak from chemo, avoid supplements that lower blood counts.

Treatment history shapes every decision. If you're on immunotherapy, ask if any adjuncts might boost or block your immune response. If radiation left a scar or digestive issues, support tissue healing with targeted nutrition (keto or carnivore diet) and hydration. For those who have had surgery, focus on recovery first—then layer in metabolic or repurposed therapies once you've rebuilt strength. People finishing chemotherapy may need to repair their gut wall, restore beneficial bacteria, and rebuild stamina before adding anything new. Your protocol will shift with each new scan, symptom, or lab result.

Cancer is never static. What you need today might shift tomorrow. The trick is staying curious and responsive. Always start from where you are—your diagnosis, your treatment history, your current labs—and keep updating as your situation evolves. There's no one recipe for everyone (aside from diet). Even though all cancers share a metabolic root, your lived experience shapes the best response for you.

As this chapter comes to a close, remember that personalization is ongoing—it's not about finding a perfect protocol once but about learning, adapting, and responding as your needs shift. The next chapter will look at mind-body tools and ways to support your whole self through every phase of treatment and healing.

Decision Tree Protocol Mapping

☑ Personalized Treatment Decision Tree

This tool is for education — discuss decisions with your healthcare provider.

STEP 1 — What Type of Cancer?

Circle all that apply:

◇ **A. Solid Tumors**

- Breast
- Lung
- Colorectal
- Prostate
- Pancreatic
- Liver
- Kidney
- Ovarian
- Cervical
- Endometrial
- Bladder
- Melanoma
- Head & neck
- Brain tumors & glioblastoma (special metabolic considerations ☑)

➡ **Go to STEP 2-A**

◇ **B. Hematologic / Blood Cancers**

- Leukemia
- Lymphoma
- Multiple myeloma
- MDS/MPN disorders

➡ **Go to STEP 2-B**

◇ **C. Rare Tumors / Unknown Primary**

- Neuroendocrine
- Sarcomas
- Mesothelioma
- Unknown primary cancers

➡ **Go to STEP 2-C**

STEP 2 — What Is Your Current Treatment Status?

☑ **Currently in treatment**

Check all that apply:

- Chemotherapy
- Radiation
- Immunotherapy
- Targeted therapy
- Hormone therapy
- Surgery scheduled or completed

➡ **Go to STEP 3-ON**

☑ **Not in treatment (watchful waiting or self-directed)**

➔ **Go to STEP 3-OFF**

STEP 3-ON — Integration With Existing Treatment

Goal: Reduce interactions + maximize synergy

Is your doctor supportive of integrative therapies?

- **YES → Go to STEP 4-Goals**
- **NO → Go to STEP 4-Goals**
  (use "Doctor Communication Scripts" chapter)

Contraindication Alerts
Avoid or delay repurposed drugs if you are:

- experiencing **severe cytopenias** (esp. in blood cancers)
- on **CYP450-dependent chemo** → require interaction check
- recovering from **major surgery** (delay metabolic stress)

☑ Safe categories to discuss with oncology:

- **Metabolic therapy** (keto, fasting adjustments)
- **Mind-body & lifestyle protocols**
- **Fenbendazole** cautiously with liver monitoring
- **Ivermectin** cautiously with neuro checks

➔ **Go to STEP 4-Goals**

STEP 3-OFF — Self-Directed or Post-Treatment

Goal: Choose supportive or aggressive adjuncts

Choose most accurate:

- **Newly diagnosed → Go to STEP 4-Goals**
- **Post-primary treatment (remission surveillance) → Go to STEP 4-Goals**
- **Exhausted standard options → Go to STEP 4-Goals**

Additional options:

- **Stronger metabolic interventions**
- **Broader repurposed drug stacking**

Go to STEP 4-Goals

STEP 4 — What Is Your Primary Treatment Goal?

Select ONE main priority (you can revisit later):

Main Goal	Best Starting Path
Shrink tumor now	**Press-Pulse Metabolic Therapy** + Repurposed drugs
Slow progression	Targeted repurposed drugs + lifestyle protocols
Improve quality of life	Mind-body + detox + symptom-targeted supplements
Prevent recurrence	Maintenance metabolic strategy + immune support
Support current conventional care	Low-interaction metabolic + supportive adjuncts

Go to STEP 5

STEP 5 — Recommended Strategy Pathways

Follow based on your STEP 1 cancer category:

☑ **Solid Tumors (A)**

Evidence-supported emphasis:

✔ Metabolic therapy (Seyfried → solid tumors = most glycolytic)
✔ Fenbendazole protocols
✔ Ivermectin for metastasis control
✔ Hyperbaric oxygen
✔ Supplement stacks: curcumin, CBD, medicinal mushrooms

🩸 Alerts

- If liver metastasis → **limit hepatotoxic stacks**
- If *unintentional* rapid weight loss → **avoid intensive fasting**

➡ Suggest Chapters:
Repurposed Drugs + Metabolic Therapy + HBOT + Supplement Stacks

---

☑ **Blood / Hematologic Cancers (B)**

Evidence-supported emphasis:

✔ Ivermectin in leukemia & lymphoma models
✔ Immune-supportive diet with clean animal proteins & low carbs
✔ Low-carb approach (but milder transitions)

🩸 Alerts

- Fenbendazole caution: **bone marrow suppression risk**
- No prolonged fasting during **active cytotoxic therapy**

➡ Suggest Chapters:
Ivermectin + Immune Support + Mind-Body Resilience

☑ Rare Tumors / Unknown Primary (C)

Evidence-supported emphasis:

✔ Personalized stacking

✔ Clinical trials review early

✔ Maximal metabolic flexibility strategies

🔥 Alerts

- Strong focus on **diagnostic clarity first**

➡ Suggest Chapters:
All "decision-support" chapters + Repurposed Drugs Overview

STEP 6 — Monitoring and Adjustment Cycle

Every 4–8 weeks, evaluate:

Measure	Improvement?	Action
Symptoms	☑ or stable	Maintain
Symptoms	🚫 new or worse	Adjust
Imaging	☑	Continue current plan
Tumor markers	☑ or neutral	Stay the course
Side effects	🚫 severe	Reduce or pause repurposed drugs
Overall function	↓	Shift toward QoL supportive path

➡ Re-enter at **STEP 4** with updated goals

📌 Quick Reference Key

☑ Encourage
🔥 Caution / Contraindication
➡ Leads to next decision point

Glossary Term	Suggested definition (short + neutral)
Metabolic Therapy	Strategies that reduce cancer fuel sources (like glucose) and boost healthy cell metabolism.
Repurposed Drugs	FDA-approved medications used *off-label* for potential anticancer effects based on research.
HBOT	Hyperbaric Oxygen Therapy — increased oxygen delivery to tissues; may support metabolic strategies.
CYP450-dependent chemo	Chemotherapy drugs processed by liver enzymes involved in many drug interactions.
Press (goes with pulse)	continuous metabolic stress
Pulse (goes with press)	targeted cyclic therapy
QoL	Quality of Life

Chapter 11
Mind-Body, Faith, and Emotional Resilience

Managing Scanxiety, Fear, and Information Overload

If you've ever caught yourself holding your breath before a medical scan or test, you're not alone. The tense anticipation before appointments, often called "scanxiety," can be just as daunting as the result itself. You might notice physical symptoms—heart pounding, shaky hands, poor sleep—as your mind races with "What if?" scenarios. This kind of fear is a natural response when so much is uncertain. It's not a sign of weakness or lack of faith; it's a human reaction to high-stakes waiting[19].

Anxiety often lingers beyond the appointment, making it tough to focus or enjoy daily life. You might replay doctor conversations, obsessively check for results, or fall into a late-night spiral of online research. The sheer amount of information—much of it conflicting—can be overwhelming, and finding trustworthy sources can feel impossible.

Grounding techniques help when anxiety spikes. One effective method is the “five senses check-in”: pause and list five things you see, four you can touch, three you hear, two you smell, and one you taste. This helps anchor you in the present, breaking the cycle of racing thoughts. Some people create calming rituals for scan days, like wearing a favorite sweater, listening to music, or bringing a friend for distraction. During appointments, don’t hesitate to ask for a moment to breathe or, if needed, step outside.

With information overload, setting boundaries is key. Taking breaks from symptom searches or limiting time spent in online groups can preserve mental well-being. Try setting a daily “research window”—perhaps 30 minutes at a designated time—then put your phone or laptop away. If certain forums or social feeds leave you more anxious, mute or avoid them temporarily. Choose information sources that offer comfort and empowerment rather than panic. Remember, it’s healthy to say, “That’s enough for now.”

Interactive Reflection: Emotional Check-In Tool

Once a week, check in with yourself: On a scale of 1–10, how anxious are you about your health today? What triggered your strongest feeling this week? Did anything—walking, chatting with a friend, turning off your phone—bring some relief? Jot down one thing that helped and one that made things harder. Over time, you may spot patterns that reveal what supports you best.

If anxiety becomes overwhelming—manifesting as panic attacks, deep exhaustion, or days of lost sleep—reach out for help. Many hospitals have counselors or social workers experienced with cancer care. Seeking support isn’t a weakness; your mental well-being is as important as any treatment plan. You don’t have to face this alone.

Practical Stress-Reduction Tools

Stress has a way of sneaking up on you, especially when you're dealing with cancer and considering different treatments. Sometimes, even when you think you're holding it together, your body gives you away—a clenched jaw, a headache that won't fade, or that tightness in your chest that feels like you're carrying a weight. I found that simple, evidence-based practices could make a real difference, even when life felt completely unmanageable. Meditation and mindfulness aren't just for yogis or monks; they're for anyone who wants to quiet the noise in their mind, even if just for a few moments. You don't need incense or a fancy cushion. Sometimes, all it takes is closing your eyes and focusing on the feeling of your breath moving in and out. Start with two minutes—notice each inhale, each exhale, and when your mind wanders (because it will), gently bring it back to the breath. Guided meditations can help if silence feels intimidating at first. There are free apps and YouTube channels with options ranging from body scans to loving-kindness meditations. It can be incredibly helpful to do a short gratitude practice at night, mentally naming three things you appreciated that day, no matter how small—like a warm mug of tea or a smile from a nurse.

Breathwork is another tool that can bring quick relief when anxiety spikes. It may sound too simple, but controlling your breath actually gives your nervous system a chance to reset. Try this: inhale slowly through your nose for four counts, hold for four, exhale through your mouth for six. Repeat a few times. You'll often notice your heart rate slowing, your shoulders dropping. This "4-4-6" method helps during tough moments, like waiting for a phone call or sitting in a crowded clinic. If you wake up at night with worry, focusing on long exhales can help shift your body out of fight-or-flight mode.

Quality sleep is more than just rest; it's when your body does much of its healing. Sleep can get disrupted by pain, medication, or worry. I struggled with insomnia off and on, sometimes finding myself wide awake at 4 a.m. with thoughts spinning. A regular bedtime routine, keeping screens out of the bedroom, avoiding heavy meals late at night, and keeping the bedroom cool all helped. I also started dimming the lights an hour before bed to signal to my body that it was time to wind down. If your mind won't shut off, jotting down your worries or a quick to-do list can help get them out of your head; this is commonly referred to as a "brain dump". For persistent insomnia, cognitive behavioral therapy for insomnia (CBT-I) can be more effective than medication and is worth exploring. Sleep isn't just about fighting fatigue—it's about giving your body, and your mind, the chance to recover and rebuild.

Grounding and Earthing: Science and Practice

When I first heard about grounding or "earthing"—the practice of making direct skin contact with the earth through grass, dirt, sand, or concrete—it sounded unusual. Yet, the concept is simple: connecting physically with the earth can calm your nervous system and help your body reset. At first, I was skeptical, but after trying it, I noticed subtle but real effects. Standing barefoot on grass in the morning gave me a sense of connection and stability, beyond my worry or diagnosis. Science has begun to investigate these claims. Early studies link grounding to reduced inflammation, regulated cortisol (the stress hormone), and improved sleep. Researchers propose that electrons absorbed from the earth may neutralize free radicals in the body, lowering inflammation and potentially aiding healing. Participants in studies often report less pain, fewer headaches, and more balanced moods after regular grounding sessions. It makes perfect sense from an evolutionary perspective. When our ancient human ancestors roamed the earth, they walked on the ground, slept on the ground, hunted and gathered on the ground. They weren't insulated from the earth like we are today with our rubber soles, houses and beds as far removed from the ground as we can get.

You don't need special circumstances to try this. When you're too tired to walk, simply sit with bare feet on grass or concrete for twenty minutes. Leaning against a tree or touching soil or grass while gardening can also work. For those who live in apartments or during colder months, grounding mats are available. These are designed to connect to the ground port of a wall outlet (the single hole; no current passes through you—they simply connect you to the earth's energy). However, I've read that the cleanest, truest ground is to connect the ground mat to a wire that runs under a door or window outside and attaches to a grounding rod inserted into the earth. That's what I do. I tried connecting a grounding wrist strap to the ground hole in an outlet and ended up with a headache for hours. Was that because of the ground hole connection? I'll never know, but using the grounding rod inserted about a foot into the earth doesn't cause a headache for me. Some people use grounding sheets at night as well. Personally, I've been sleeping much more deeply since adding a grounding sheet to my bed. While research is still evolving, many people—especially in cancer support circles—report feeling calmer and sleeping better with regular grounding.

Sunlight is another simple, powerful tool. Safe sun exposure boosts vitamin D, which is essential for immune health, mood, and resilience—especially important during treatment. Even ten minutes outdoors, with skin exposed to the sun, can noticeably lift mood and energy for the day. Sunlight also helps set your circadian rhythm, so getting outdoors early, even on a cloudy day, can make a difference in nighttime sleep. During my morning barefoot grounding on my lawn, I turn my closed eyes toward the sun for 30 seconds to help reset or reconfirm my circadian rhythm.

Harnessing Faith and Spirituality

Faith has long been a foundation in my life, but it was truly tested when loved ones battled cancer. During those toughest days, faith became more than belief in a higher power—it was hope amid chaos. For many, faith offers comfort, purpose, and strength when fear and sadness feel overwhelming. Even a simple repeated prayer during treatment or whispered before sleep makes uncertainty feel less heavy. Faith isn't about having answers; sometimes it's just trusting you're not facing this alone, that something greater is with you through the struggle, sharing your burdens.

Deepening a spiritual connection doesn't require strict practices or constant attendance at services. I found peace in quiet ways: reading favorite passages, lighting a candle, or walking outdoors and talking to God—or whatever resonates with you. Sometimes, music or poetry speak for people when they can't find the words. Others find ritual comforting—using meditation beads, journaling prayers, or sitting in silence honoring small moments of gratitude. If faith feels distant, that's okay. Spirituality might appear in awe at a sunrise or the warmth of shared laughter. Leaning into familiar prayers or traditions can bring structure and comfort, while those without a formal faith can find peace and connection through nature, loved ones, or the universe.

Pastoral counseling and spiritual support groups can help when things become too heavy. Pastors, chaplains, and spiritual counselors can sit with pain without trying to fix it, allowing space to voice fears and doubts. Group settings—whether church-based or interfaith—can help you know you're not alone in your struggles. Simply hearing "I'm scared too" from someone else could bring comfort. Many hospitals and cancer centers offer spiritual care regardless of religious affiliation. Chaplains are trained to support people of any or no faith.

Discussing spiritual needs with your care team can feel vulnerable, but it helps you be seen as a whole person, not just a diagnosis. Learn to say, "My faith is important to me," or "I'd like prayer as part of my treatment." Some medical professionals engage easily in these conversations; others may not know how to respond, but expressing your needs is still worthwhile. If you want prayer before a procedure or time for a ritual, ask for it—your beliefs deserve respect. Even if your care team doesn't share your faith, they can help create space for what matters most to you. And if you aren't sure whether it will help, there's one way to find out; it may surprise you.

Building Your Support Network

After cancer struck my family, I quickly learned that isolation makes everything harder. The shock of diagnosis, exhausting appointments, and anxiety become much heavier when faced alone. Genuine connection with others who understand what you are going through, or peer support, isn't necessarily about sharing medical tips, but real conversation, shared laughter, and having a space to vent, cry, or just be honest. Sometimes, one empathetic comment from someone who "gets it" can break through days of anxiety better than anything a doctor might say. You might connect with others who share your diagnosis or those in similar circumstances, finding common ground in shared fears, hopes, and experiences.

There's an abundance of online support groups. Some Facebook communities are positive and well-moderated, offering practical advice and encouragement. Others, by contrast, can seem chaotic, filled with misinformation or negativity. Over time, you learn to seek out groups with clear guidelines, active moderation, and a healthy balance of optimism and honesty. Sites like Inspire and Reddit also offer smaller forums focused on specific cancer types or care perspectives. Reading posts before participating helps gauge a group's tone. Never hesitate to leave a group if it drains you—your emotional energy is limited, so invest it wisely.

Online connections can be invaluable, yet there's a unique comfort in meeting face-to-face. Local hospitals, cancer centers, and community organizations often run support circles or host educational gatherings. Even a small coffee meet-up with others going through similar experiences can make a difference. Finding these groups might require persistence—check flyers at clinics, talk with nurses, or look on community boards at libraries, community centers, or local online news websites. In-person connections bring warmth and trust that's hard to replicate online. Sometimes, a glance or a hug conveys support words can't.

Creating a balanced support network takes intention. Though it's easy to get swept up in discussions about cancer, it's important to include friends, family, or groups who help you focus on life beyond illness. People who chat about books, movies, or the weather give you a break from the constant medical focus. Nurturing relationships can bring lightness to all your days, not just those centered around treatment. That balance—connections with people who understand cancer and those who bring unrelated joys—can help you feel like a whole person, not just a patient or caregiver. Asking for and accepting help isn't always easy, but it can be transformative. Often, the most healing conversations are the simple, unexpected ones—moments that remind you you're still yourself, supported by others.

Caregiver Strategies

Caring for someone with cancer is a role few are prepared for. Suddenly, you're managing medications, appointments, and paperwork, while also striving to provide hope and stability. The emotional toll can be immense, with caregivers often feeling invisible, their needs put aside by the urgency of their loved one's illness. Caregivers become the steady backbone of the household, holding everything together despite exhaustion. The challenge is not just physical tasks, but also the mental load: remembering medication schedules, monitoring symptoms, and dealing with the rollercoaster of emotions brought on by every medical update. Feelings of guilt for being overwhelmed or wanting time alone are normal. Caregivers face their own, often unspoken, struggles.

Listening and Support

Offering effective support means listening deeply, rather than trying to fix every problem. Sometimes, your loved one just needs your quiet presence or a listening ear for their fears and frustrations. Small gestures—bringing water, preparing a favorite meal, or jotting down questions for the doctor—often mean more than elaborate plans or advice. There's no need to be perfect or have all the answers. It's okay to admit, "I'm not sure, but I'll find out," or simply, "I'm here for you." Being present, even in uncertain moments, is a profound act of care.

Self-Care and Boundaries

Self-care for caregivers is essential, not selfish. Burnout happens if you never take breaks. Short pauses—a walk, coffee with a friend, or reading—replenish energy and patience. Setting boundaries, though uncomfortable at first, is necessary to sustain the ability to care. Saying, "I need some time for myself," is healthy and protects your long-term capacity to help.

Delegating tasks or accepting help, even if others do things differently, reduces emotional strain and resentment.

Communication and Appreciation

Open, honest communication keeps care partnerships strong. Discussing needs, limits, and fears on both sides prevents misunderstandings. Regular check-ins about what's working and what's not can head off larger conflicts. Using a shared notebook or calendar for appointments and medicines can help everyone stay organized and lighten the mental burden. Simple thanks or kind notes can make tough days brighter.

Caregiving, though difficult, can create deep bonds and unexpected moments of closeness and gratitude. Recognizing both the hardships and the joys allows for genuine connection. Remember: your role matters, not because you're perfect, but because you show up with care and honesty. In the next chapter, we'll explore resources and ongoing learning to support both patients and caregivers as you continue this journey of healing and hope.

Chapter 12
Resources, Research, and Ongoing Learning

Understanding and Participating in Clinical Trials

Cancer research often feels both fast-moving and painfully slow. Clinical trials are where new treatments become real possibilities. Whether you're cautious or curious, understanding clinical trials can give you more control and confidence in your care options. It's important to know how to find them, what they involve, and whether one might be right for you.

Clinical trials may sound intimidating, but they are carefully organized studies meant to improve or test new treatments—or look at new ways to use known therapies. Every medicine in use today was once a clinical trial. Trials vary: some test new drugs, others explore different combinations, dosages, or supportive care. You might notice terms like "randomized," "placebo-controlled," or "open-label." Don't let jargon put you off. The main aim is to find what works best and is safest for real people.

An explanation of trials continues below, but it's important to understand what a "new drug" might mean. It costs billions of dollars to research, trial, get FDA approval, and bring a new drug to the market, whether for cancer or anything else. Because of this, drug developers will often slightly tweak an old drug (sometimes just by changing one molecule) so it can be legally be called a new drug. This information is not to dishearten you, but to enlighten you. Oncology research continues to try to prove that cancer is a genetic disease despite increasing metabolic evidence. So drug development continues down this mostly meaningless path. I say mostly, because a "new" drug might actually help 4% of the patients using it. Ok, back to trials.

Trials move through different phases. Phase I is the first test in people—usually a small group focused on safety and dosage. Often, these are for those who've run out of standard options, but sometimes others are eligible. Phase II trials are larger, studying whether the treatment has real effects—like shrinking tumors, slowing disease, or improving quality of life. Phase III trials are big—often hundreds or thousands of patients across hospitals or countries—comparing the new approach to today's standard of care. These trials often decide if a new therapy becomes the new "normal." Phase IV occurs after a treatment is approved, watching for long-term or rare side effects.

How do you find a trial? It can seem overwhelming but your oncologist is the best starting point—they may know of trials that fit your diagnosis and situation. If they don't mention it, ask directly. You can also consider second opinions or contact major cancer centers. The National Cancer Institute's (NCI) Cancer Information Service (1-800-4-CANCER) has people who'll help you search for relevant trials. Online, try the NCI's clinical trial search or clinicaltrials.gov; you'll need to enter information like your cancer type, stage, previous treatments, and genetic results—these details influence eligibility.

When you spot a trial, don't rush. The summaries are often full of complex language—go slowly, and jot down questions. Check for: what treatments are being tested, how many appointments are needed, what scans or tests you'd need, any costs or covered expenses. Write everything down—small details matter.

If you want to apply, usually you or your doctor contact the research team (info is always listed). The next step is "screening"—checking your medical history, lab results, and more to see if you match "eligibility" requirements. Criteria are often strict—based on diagnosis, prior therapies, lab numbers, age, other conditions, or genetic factors.

Joining a clinical trial means following a detailed plan, or protocol. You'll probably have more office visits and tests than in standard care, including extra scans, labs, and questionnaires. Some find this close monitoring reassuring; others find it tiring. It's important to ask about time and travel demands up front. You'll have a study nurse or coordinator as your main contact. And you can leave any study at any time for any reason.

There are real trade-offs. The positives: access to new therapies, the chance to help future patients, and sometimes more personalized support, such as extra monitoring or travel help. On the other hand, new treatments may not work better than what's already available and could have unexpected side effects. Some trials randomize participants, meaning you might get standard treatment or a placebo, depending on the trial design.

Ethics are strict. Before anything begins, you must go through "informed consent"—the research team explains risks and benefits in plain language and answers all your questions. Never feel rushed or pressured. If you're uncomfortable or questions aren't answered honestly, it's okay to step back.

Interactive Element: Clinical Trial Reflection Worksheet

Before you decide, take ten minutes with this reflection:

- What are my top three hopes for being in a trial?
- What's my biggest worry?

- Do I understand what happens if I join—or if I don't?
- Who can I talk to for honest advice (doctor, family, friend)?
- What practical issues might make a difference (travel, time off, child care)?
- What questions do I still have?

Write down your answers and take them to your next conversation with your doctor or the research team. This is about your life—use this tool to make sure your choice is right for you.

Being informed about clinical trials doesn't require joining one. It means you have choices, and those choices bring hope in uncertain times.

Top Patient Forums, Advocacy Groups, and Continuing Education

When you first seek practical knowledge outside your doctor's office, it can feel isolating. But there's actually a vast network of people sharing what helps, what hurts, and what's just hype. Online patient forums are lifelines for many dealing with cancer, offering a real sense of connection and honest conversation. The most active communities can be found on Inspire, CancerCompass, Smart Patients, and Reddit's r/cancer. Searching terms like "fenbendazole cancer forum," "alternative cancer protocol," or "metabolic therapy group" reveals threads where people openly discuss doses, side effects, brands, victories, setbacks, and daily struggles. Some provide credible details, lab results, and photos, while others offer practical tips or simply seek support. Each forum has a unique vibe—some are science-heavy, others blend hope and personal stories. It's best to read silently at first to gauge the tone and identify trustworthy voices. If you join in, consider protecting your privacy: use a nickname, avoid sharing personal details, and be thoughtful about what you post.

Beyond message boards, advocacy groups give structure and power to the push for better treatments and patient rights. These organizations are vibrant communities, not just websites. The American Cancer Society, for instance, provides support lines, local events, and trained navigators who can help with everything from insurance to emotional support. Other resources like CancerCare[20] offer free emotional and practical support, support groups (both online and in-person), and education for patients and caregivers.

If metabolic or integrative oncology interests you, explore the **Foundation for Metabolic Cancer Therapies**[21], which contains a lot of education. The **Society for Integrative Oncology**[22] and the **Metabolic Terrain Institute of Health**[23] link you to research, practitioners, and a like-minded community. For rare or specific cancers, groups like the Multiple Myeloma Research Foundation or the Pancreatic Cancer Action Network can provide specialized info, clinical trial updates, and sometimes even financial aid for travel or treatments. These advocacy groups often drive research into repurposed drugs or new therapies, sometimes even funding studies larger organizations overlook. Their newsletters and webinars are treasure troves of current information.

Keeping your knowledge current is important, since cancer research changes rapidly. Webinars and podcasts often provide more insight than hospital handouts. The **Association of Cancer Care Centers**[24] hosts webinars on new treatments, side effect management, and patient advocacy; many are open to patients seeking to ask smarter questions and better understand their options. Podcasts like "**Cancer Straight Talk from MSK** (Memorial Sloan Kettering)[25]." Most advocacy groups also offer regular online events with Q&As, covering everything from metabolic diet strategies to mind-body techniques. Don't dismiss local hospital workshops or public library talks—they often deliver the most practical tips on stress, nutrition (if it's plant-based, take it with a grain of salt), or legal rights.

Online courses help you go deeper on your schedule. Sites like Coursera and edX have free classes on topics like cancer biology, nutrition, and clinical trials; auditing is usually free without a certificate. Many big cancer centers offer hands-on workshops on cooking for specific diets, meditation, or record organization. Start with one resource at a time; trying to keep up with everything is overwhelming. Bookmark what you find most helpful, unsubscribe if something feels like too much, and revisit trusted sources regularly.

Navigating Information and Staying Safe

Being active online demands discernment. Not every friendly poster is credible, and opinion often gets mixed with fact. Watch out for miracle cure claims and aggressive product pitches.

The best online spaces allow honest disagreement and nuanced discussion. If a group suppresses reasonable questions or deletes posts about side effects, be wary. Healthy communities talk about both successes and failures and admit when things go wrong. Often, the most valuable support comes from those willing to listen, not just lecture. Sometimes, seeing someone else's tough day described honestly can make your own feel less lonely.

Getting Started

If you're new to all this, try these steps:

1. Pick one forum and read through recent threads on topics that interest you.
2. Sign up for a newsletter from an advocacy group that aligns with your needs.
3. Listen to a podcast episode while commuting or doing chores.
4. Watch a webinar (live or recorded) on a topic you want to learn more about.

Connecting with others who "get it" can be incredibly comforting and practical. Whether you learn a new tip for managing side effects, hear about research into alternative protocols, or just find reassurance that you're not facing cancer alone, these resources can lighten difficult days. You don't have to become an expert overnight, but staying informed gives you a louder voice in your care—and sometimes even a little hope when things feel heavy.

How to Spot and Avoid Scams, Hype, and Outdated Protocols

After what my family went through with cancer, I became acutely aware of how easy it is to fall for hype when hope is scarce. The sheer number of "miracle cure" ads, secret protocols, and bold promises online is overwhelming—and can be dangerous. And, unless you search in a private browser window (like Chrome incognito) you'll see a sudden onslaught of relevant ads; so just be aware of this.

Be cautious with money-back guarantees and glowing testimonials, especially if the photos seem staged or generic. Legitimate treatments don't need persuasive marketing or testimonials that sound too perfect.

Cancer—and the human body—are complex. Scams exploit desperation, preying on people by creating urgency ("limited supply," countdown timers, pressuring you to buy now). If you're being told time is running out, be wary. Fear and urgency can cloud judgment.

Now, I approach supposed new protocols or products like a detective. Who's making the claim? Often, it's someone with no medical or research credentials—just a flashy website and unverifiable stories. Look for real contact information, a physical address, and independent reviews. If you can't determine who runs the site or where the company is located, that's a warning sign. Also, consider what else they're selling. Are they directing you to buy supplements, private coaching, or "exclusive" products? Genuine doctors and researchers share their findings without pressuring you to purchase.

Another tactic is excessive technical jargon meant to impress rather than inform. I've seen many sites throw around terms like "epigenetic modulation," "quantum healing," or "DNA repair" without clear, plain explanations. When information is hidden under buzzwords or you're told you won't understand unless you're a scientist, it's likely there's nothing substantial being offered.

When I evaluate a new protocol, my process is straightforward. I search for published studies, ideally in medical journals or trusted scientific sources, and check for real scientists or doctors with verifiable credentials. Also, look at who funded the research. If it's from a supplement company or anyone likely to profit, be extra skeptical—financial interests can bias research. One small or old study, never repeated elsewhere, isn't good evidence.

Check whether reputable cancer centers, universities, or respected patient organizations discuss the protocol. If it only appears on forums or on sites selling the product, that's a red flag. For older therapies, check when the last studies were published—medical science evolves quickly. Outdated advice can be not only ineffective but also dangerous, especially if it interferes with current treatments.

Following outdated or debunked protocols poses real risks. Some once-promising treatments have later been proven ineffective or even harmful. Sometimes these protocols interact negatively with real medications.

Scam and Protocol Evaluation Checklist

- Is there credible, peer-reviewed research—or just anecdotes?
- Does a respected cancer center, or cancer researcher, discuss this?
- Who is making the claim, and are they qualified?
- Who funded the research, and do they profit if you buy?
- Are there warnings from trustworthy groups about risks?
- Does the product or protocol use miracle language?
- Are you pressured to buy or discouraged from consulting your doctor?

If the last two get a "yes" or the first two get a "no," it's time to step back.

It's understandable to want hope, especially when options feel scarce. It's okay to hope—just match hope with caution and be diligent about asking questions. Accurate information protects both your wallet and your health. Always talk openly with your care team about new protocols, even if you fear judgment—their priority is your safety.

Sorting fact from fiction isn't about crushing hope, but about making space for real, helpful options by tuning out the noise. Protecting yourself from scams and outdated ideas lets you focus on genuine support and effective choices.

In closing, remember that asking questions and staying alert protects your health as much as any supplement or therapy. The next section will guide you in building a protocol tailored to your unique needs and goals, helping you move ahead with clarity and confidence.

Chapter 13
Rapid-Fire Questions: Clarity, Confidence, and Action

Have you ever found yourself staring at the ceiling at three in the morning, your mind racing with every question that's piled up since the diagnosis, hoping for that one clear answer that would make things less frightening?. Sometimes it feels like every bit of advice only sparks more confusion—especially when the stakes are this high. So in this chapter, I want to give you something different: straight-up clarity. This is where we cut through the clutter and tackle those burning questions you wish you could ask your oncologist, nutritionist, or that person who always seems to "know someone who beat cancer doing X." Each answer is brief, direct, and points you to the right spot in this book if you want to dig deeper. No fluff, just facts and honest guidance to help you move forward without getting lost in the weeds.

How do I know if a repurposed drug is right for me?

Choosing to add any repurposed drug—whether it's fenbendazole, ivermectin, or something else—starts with knowing your own story. Consider your diagnosis, stage, current treatments, and overall health. Are you already on chemo or radiation? Are you looking for gentler options because standard care isn't tolerable or effective? If you're still in active treatment, it's vital to talk through your plans with your oncology team. But if you've reached a point where standard options are exhausted or simply not right for you, repurposed drugs can be appealing. Ask yourself what you hope to achieve—tumor shrinkage, slowing progression, better quality of life? If your answer is yes to any of those, and you've got a reasonable safety net (a supportive doctor or at least frequent lab monitoring), then exploring repurposed drugs could make sense for you. See Chapter 6 and Chapter 7 for side-by-side comparisons and sourcing tips.

What's the real risk of side effects or toxicity with these drugs?

Risks vary by drug and by your own unique body. Fenbendazole generally causes mild digestive upset if anything; ivermectin can trigger dizziness or rashes in some people. Mebendazole is usually easy on the system but can irritate the liver if taken long-term. Nitazoxanide sometimes leads to an upset stomach or harmless orange urine. The real danger often comes from stacking too many therapies at once or ignoring early warning signs—like yellowing skin, odd bruising, confusion, or severe headaches. Get baseline labs (liver enzymes, kidney function, blood counts) before starting anything new, then recheck every few weeks. If you notice any major change in energy, mood, or physical symptoms that last more than a few days (or get worse), stop the new agent and call your doctor. For a full rundown of side effects and red flags, see Chapter 9.

How do I avoid dangerous drug interactions?

Start by listing every prescription, supplement, and over-the-counter medication you take. Include vitamins, herbal teas, even those "occasional" ibuprofen tablets. Cross-check for known interactions—especially liver-metabolized drugs like many chemotherapies (they use enzymes like CYP3A4 or CYP2C19). If you don't know where to start, websites like Drugs.com have interaction checkers, but nothing beats a pharmacist's input. When adding a new repurposed drug, introduce it alone for a week or two before stacking others. If you're taking chemo or immunotherapy concurrently, ask your oncologist about potential overlaps—even if they're skeptical about your alternative protocol. Documentation is your friend here; keep notes on everything taken and how you feel each day. See Chapter 9 for a more detailed breakdown.

Can I combine more than one repurposed drug at a time?

Yes—but do so cautiously. Combining fenbendazole and ivermectin (or adding in mebendazole or nitazoxanide) isn't unheard of, and some people feel stacking gives them a better shot at hitting cancer from multiple angles. The safest way is to start with one agent at the lowest effective dose. Wait two weeks before adding another. Monitor yourself closely for side effects and review lab results regularly. Avoid stacking drugs with the same mechanism (like fenbendazole and mebendazole) unless under medical supervision, since they both stress the liver. Keep hydration up and support your liver with a healthy diet and rest. If you ever feel overwhelmed by symptoms or see labs trending badly (rising bilirubin, dropping white counts), scale back immediately and consult your doctor or pharmacist. See Chapter 6 for sample stacks and Chapter 10 for customization ideas.

Is there any way to know if these protocols are working for me?

Objective tracking is key—you can't trust only how you feel day to day because cancer can be sneaky. Use tumor markers (like PSA (prostate), CA-125 (ovarian), CEA (colorectal/pancreatic), AFP (liver), and CA 15-3/CA 27.29 (breast)), imaging (CT, PET, MRI), and blood tests to gauge progress every few months (or as often as your insurance allows). Keep a journal of symptoms: note energy levels, pain scores, sleep quality, appetite changes, new side effects, mood shifts—these can sometimes reveal subtle improvements or problems before labs do. Don't ignore gut feelings either; if something feels off or different in a good way, make a note. Over time, patterns will emerge that help guide next steps (adjusting doses, switching protocols, or stopping something that isn't helping). Check Chapter 9 and 10 for tracking templates and more on monitoring progress.

Where should I actually buy these drugs and supplements?

Quality matters more than price or convenience here. For human-grade medications like ivermectin or mebendazole, use licensed pharmacies whenever possible—even if it means getting a prescription from an integrative doctor or via telemedicine. For veterinary drugs like fenbendazole (Panacur C is a common brand), stick with reputable pet supply outlets that provide batch numbers and certificates of analysis. Check every COA yourself—make sure it matches your lot number and shows testing for purity and contaminants. Avoid anything with vague origins or no customer service number; scams are rampant online. For supplements (curcumin, CBD oil), pick brands that use third-party testing and transparent labeling—don't buy bulk powders from unknown sellers on auction sites. Chapter 6 offers step-by-step sourcing checklists, and an explanation of a COA. Resources shows a sample COA.

How do I calculate dosing for these medications?

Dosing depends on both the drug and your weight/health status. Fenbendazole: most adults use 222 mg per day (one packet of Panacur C), three days on/four days off (the "Joe Tippens protocol"). Ivermectin: dosing is weight-based—0.2 mg/kg per day is typical for adults (so a 70 kg person would take about 14 mg), sometimes split into two smaller doses per day. Mebendazole: often 100–200 mg twice daily. Nitazoxanide: usually 500 mg twice daily with food. Always start low if sensitive or frail; titrate upward only if tolerated well after one to two weeks. Never double up after missed doses; just resume as scheduled. Always round doses down rather than up unless supervised by a doctor. Chapter 4 and 5 have more complete dosing guides.

What if I miss a dose?

Don't panic—missing one dose won't undo weeks of progress. If it's only been a few hours since your scheduled time, take it as soon as you remember unless it's almost time for the next dose (then skip it). Never double up doses to "catch up." Mark it in your medication log so you can track if this happens often—if so, consider setting reminders on your phone or using a pill organizer to keep things easier to manage when days get hectic or stressful.

Will insurance cover any of these therapies?

Almost never for repurposed drugs used off-label or veterinary formulations—unless you have a doctor who can justify their use for another approved condition (like treating parasites). Some supplements might be covered with flexible spending accounts (FSA/HSA), but most are out-of-pocket expenses. To avoid surprises, call your insurer before starting anything expensive; ask about prior authorizations for extra bloodwork or imaging related to alternative therapies as well. If you're struggling financially, reach out to advocacy groups or hospital social workers—many can help navigate grants or patient assistance programs even if traditional coverage doesn't apply.

What do I do if my family or doctor thinks I'm making a mistake?

This might be one of the toughest situations—feeling isolated when all you want is support. Start with honest communication: share why you're considering these options (hope for better quality of life, fewer side effects, more control). Show them this book, print out relevant research studies, or send them to Foundation For Metabolic Cancer Therapies at https://foundationformetaboliccancertherapies.com/metabolic-theory-of-cancer/ so they see it isn't just "something off the internet." (There's a lot of educational material there you would probably enjoy as well.) Remind everyone that you're not necessarily rejecting conventional care—you're just trying to make informed choices that fit your values and situation. Offer regular updates so loved ones don't feel left out; invite them to appointments or support groups if they're open to it. If a doctor dismisses you outright without discussion, consider seeking another opinion from an integrative provider who will meet you where you are instead of shutting down conversation.

Can I change my protocol mid-stream if something isn't working?

Absolutely—and you should! Protocols aren't written in stone; flexibility keeps you safe and responsive to what your body is telling you. If labs worsen, new side effects develop, or symptoms change unexpectedly (for better or worse), it's okay to step back and reassess. Drop one drug at a time rather than several at once so you know what's actually responsible for any changes. Keep tracking everything in writing so patterns become obvious over time—a symptom diary is worth its weight in gold here.

How do I decide when enough is enough?

This question has haunted me more than once—watching my brother struggle through treatments that left him feeling worse than the disease itself made me realize there's no single "right" answer here. It comes down to listening to your body (and your spirit), checking in with trusted supporters (friends, faith leaders, medical providers), and being honest about what matters most to you now. Longevity at any cost? Comfort? Time with family? There's courage in stepping back when treatments no longer serve those goals—and there's no shame in choosing peace over pushing forward just because others expect it.

Are there any warning signs that mean I should stop immediately?

Yes—certain symptoms mean STOP right away: sudden severe abdominal pain; yellowing eyes/skin; unexplained bruising/bleeding; confusion; loss of consciousness; persistent vomiting; chest pain; new neurological symptoms like vision changes or slurred speech; unexplained high fever or chills lasting more than a day. These can signal organ failure, infection, blood clots—or other life-threatening issues that need urgent medical attention regardless of what protocol you're on.

Do dietary changes really make much difference if I'm already on medication?

The right nutrition can create an environment where therapies work better—and where your body can recover between treatments instead of being battered nonstop by side effects. Evidence shows that metabolic therapies, like a ketogenic or carnivore diet, can not only slow tumor growth, but also reduce inflammation and support immune function. Eliminating sugars/starches and highly processed foods, adding healthy fats, prioritizing protein and fat can improve energy and resilience over time. You don't have to go all-in overnight; gradual shifts are more sustainable and less overwhelming. Chapter 2 provides a detailed look at metabolic therapies including diet.

Should I avoid all carbs or go zero-carb/carnivore?

Strict carb restriction fuels ketosis and stresses cancer cells metabolically. My research indicates it is beneficial to eat as low-carb as you can—not just to stress cancer cells, but to nourish and energize your body. Start by eliminating obvious junk foods/sugars/starches first—these inarguably serve no nutritive purpose. Over the next week or two, eliminate grains: breads, pasta, cereals. Over the following week or two eliminate high-carb vegetables. Then eliminate high-carb fruits over the following week or two. Chapter 2 gives a detailed explanation of keto/carnivore diets.

Is there any point using grounding/earthing as part of my wellness routine?

It may sound "woo" at first glance but growing evidence supports grounding as a gentle way to reduce inflammation and support sleep[26]. Even five minutes barefoot on grass each day can help regulate mood and calm frazzled nerves—not a cure for cancer but part of an overall strategy for keeping stress hormones down and healing up. Grounding sheets or mats are also effective, especially if bypassing household electrical grounding outlets and wiring these directly to a metal rod driven into the earth outside a door or window, which can easily accommodate the very thin wire and still close properly.

How can I protect myself from fake medicines online?

Vigilance is non-negotiable here! Buying from sources providing batch numbers and independent COAs showing purity testing is ideal. At the very least, look for a GMP Certification:

- Manufactured in facilities that follow Good Manufacturing Practice standards Quality Control

You may also see language like:

- Multi-stage testing for batch accuracy and consistency, secure packaging
- Each batch is sealed to preserve freshness and integrity.

The product listing shows it's manufactured under strict quality control standards. Avoid sellers with vague contact info or aggressive marketing ("miracle cure" banners). Scrutinize packaging: spelling errors, generic white bottles with stick-on labels? Major red flag! Check customer reviews for depth—not just five stars but detailed stories of real experiences. When in doubt, ask pharmacists or patient communities for vetted supplier lists before buying anything new.

Do I need a prescription for these drugs?

For human-grade ivermectin and mebendazole: yes—a prescription is legally required in most countries. In the United States, four states have recently passed laws authorizing ivermectin for human use[27], which may help ease concerns your doctor may have. Veterinary fenbendazole:

typically available over-the-counter at pet stores but not intended for human use (so quality standards vary). Nitazoxanide usually requires a prescription as well. Some telemedicine providers may be open to discussing off-label options if presented with research supporting your case[28].

What's the difference between "off-label" use and illegal use?

"Off-label" means using an approved drug for an unapproved condition—a common practice in oncology when evidence supports safety/effectiveness. Illegal use usually refers to importing unregulated substances without prescriptions or buying/selling controlled meds outside legal channels. Always document everything thoroughly if self-treating; consult legal/medical professionals if unsure about local laws.

How frequently should I get labs done while on these protocols?

Every situation differs but most people should get baseline bloodwork before starting anything new (liver enzymes, kidney function, blood counts). After starting an alternative protocol: recheck every 2–4 weeks at first; then space out if things remain stable. Any sudden symptom change? Get labs sooner rather than later.

Can I travel while using alternative protocols?

Travel is possible—but plan ahead! Carry meds/supplements in original packaging with batch numbers/prescriptions handy in case customs has questions. Bring enough supply plus extras for delays; pack copies of all relevant medical records (including recent labs/scans) on paper AND saved digitally on your phone/cloud storage. Consider time zone changes when scheduling doses—set alarms as reminders.

Are there any supplements I should definitely avoid?

Some supplements interact dangerously with chemo/radiation: garlic, ginkgo, echinacea, St John's wort (affects liver metabolism), grapefruit extract (alters drug absorption), even green tea extract interfere with the drug bortezomid/Velcade), plus anything that thins blood excessively (high-dose fish oil) without guidance[29]. When in doubt—ask your pharmacist!

Do these protocols work for all cancer types?

No single protocol looks exactly the same for every person, but this does not mean that different cancers lack a shared weakness. Research led by Thomas Seyfried and others describes cancer as a **metabolic disease**, meaning that cancer cells have damaged energy systems and rely on fermentation—using fuels like glucose and, in many cases, glutamine—to survive. From this perspective, all cancers depend on altered energy metabolism, even though how that dependency shows up can differ from person to person.

When metabolic approaches appear to "work better" for some cancers than others, the issue is usually **how the therapy is applied**, not the type of cancer itself. Strategies that focus only on lowering glucose may leave as glutamine untouched, allowing cancer cells to adapt. This can create the impression that certain cancers are less responsive, when in reality the underlying metabolic vulnerability is still present. For this reason, metabolic therapy and repurposed drugs are best used as part of a **thoughtful, adaptable plan**, rather than as one-size-fits-all solutions. Individual tolerance, safety, and real-world experience matter—and claims of universal cures should always be viewed with caution.

What's the deal with "press-pulse" therapy? Is it worth trying?

No single protocol looks exactly the same for every person, but this does not mean that different cancers lack a shared weakness. Thomas Seyfried and others describe cancer as a **metabolic disease**, meaning that cancer cells have damaged energy systems and rely on fermentation—using fuels like glucose and, in many cases, glutamine—to survive. From this perspective, all cancers depend on altered energy metabolism, even though how that dependency shows up can differ from person to person.

When metabolic approaches appear to "work better" for some cancers than others, the issue is usually **how the therapy is applied**, not the type of cancer itself. Strategies that focus only on lowering glucose may leave another fuel source—such as glutamine—untouched, allowing cancer cells to adapt. This can create the impression that certain cancers are less responsive, when in reality the underlying metabolic vulnerability is still present. For this reason, metabolic therapy and repurposed drugs are best used as part of a **thoughtful, adaptable plan**, rather than as one-size-fits-all solutions. Individual tolerance, safety, and real-world experience matter—and claims of universal cures should always be viewed with caution.

When do I need professional help adjusting my protocol?

You should reach out anytime labs worsen unexpectedly; new side effects persist beyond three days; confusion/memory lapses emerge suddenly; energy nosedives without explanation; pain spikes unmanageable levels; sleep completely unravels despite self-care efforts; OR when considering stacking multiple agents/adding anything unfamiliar.

Interactive Tool: Personalized Protocol Audit

Take out paper and write down every medication/supplement currently used (dose/time/reason). Next to each entry:

- Mark if it's supported by human studies.
- List last date labs were checked.
- Note any recent symptoms/side effects.
- Rate energy/sleep/mood from 1-10.

- Circle anything added in past month.
- Star items discussed with your provider.
- Draw arrows for suspected interactions.
- Ask: What can be simplified? What needs monitoring soon? Where could help be needed?
- Commit to bringing this sheet to every appointment—for collaborative adjustments!

This quick audit often uncovers easy fixes—missed doses, forgotten supplements causing issues—or points where simplification brings relief.

Is there anyone who shouldn't try these protocols?

Pregnant/breastfeeding women should exercise extreme caution when considering experimental regimens due to unknown risks. Those with severe liver/kidney failure[30] need strict medical supervision—or may need to avoid entirely. Consult your integrative medical professional for personalized advice[31]. People unable to log symptoms/take meds accurately without support may be at higher risk for mistakes/harm.

Are there any clinical trials on these therapies?

A growing number—but most are early-stage pilot studies rather than large-scale randomized trials[32]. Major academic centers are now running trials combining metabolic diets with standard care; some smaller studies focus on repurposed drugs alone or stacked with other agents. Search clinicaltrials.gov by cancer type + agent name—or ask at major cancer centers about ongoing studies.

If my cancer returns after remission, can I restart these protocols?

Often yes—with adjustments based on current health/lab status. Some people resume earlier regimens after recurrence while others switch up agents based on what worked previously versus what might fit now. Always get updated scans/labs before restarting anything significant.

What should caregivers focus on most?

Support comes down to listening without fixing; helping organize meds/appointments; tracking symptoms together; offering breaks from cancer talk when needed; protecting their own rest/nutrition/social life so burnout doesn't steal hope from both sides. Encourage shared routines that bring normalcy—a favorite show at night, short walks together—even during tough spells.

Do alternative protocols work right away?

Rarely! Most people notice subtle shifts in energy/sleep/appetite within weeks but significant tumor changes can take months (if they happen). Consistency matters more than intensity—steady routines beat bursts of unsustainable effort every time.

Can I use these protocols alongside palliative/hospice care?

Yes—and many find integrative approaches ease pain/nausea/anxiety while respecting comfort goals. Be open about all therapies used so care teams can coordinate symptom management safely.

Should I share my protocol details online?

It helps others—but protect privacy! Share only what feels safe; avoid posting full names/addresses/batch numbers publicly; consider using private or closed groups/forums vetted by advocacy organizations.

What do I say when friends offer unsolicited advice?

Thank them kindly—then set boundaries as needed ("I appreciate that suggestion—I'll check it out later" or "Right now my plan is working for me"). Not every tip needs following up!

Can children/teens use these approaches too?

Protocols covered here are based on adult data—with rare exceptions for older teens under strict medical supervision. Children's bodies process drugs differently so pediatric oncologist input is always needed first.

How do I keep hope alive during setbacks?

Focus on small wins: one good meal/day without pain/deep conversation/a night's sleep—all count as victories worth celebrating alongside big milestones.

Does faith/spirituality really help healing outcomes?

Research shows spiritual practices improve mental health/resilience—even physical outcomes—in serious illness. I know it helps for my family and me. Whatever brings comfort, be it prayer/meditation/nature walks/scripture—it's all valid. A study by Dr. Andrew Newberg indicates that at least 12 minutes of daily prayer or meditation can slow age-related brain decline and reduce activity in areas of the brain associated with fear, anxiety, and depression[33].

Can I still work/socialize while using these protocols?

Yes—with planning! Communicate honestly about needs/energy swings; schedule rest breaks into workdays/social events; don't hesitate to ask for flexibility around appointments/treatments.

Who do I call if things spiral out of control emotionally?

Don't wait until crisis hits—reach out early! Trusted friends/family/counselors/spiritual guides/hotlines/hospital social workers—all are equipped to listen/support/jump into action as needed.

Is there ever such thing as too much information?

Absolutely! Set limits on research time; pick a few trustworthy sources instead of endless searching; trust your gut when overload strikes—it's okay to tune out sometimes for mental peace.

Are there silver bullets—or just lots of little steps?

There are no magic cures—but stacking many small habits/interventions adds up over time: better food/sleep/movement/stress-relief/support/protocol tweaks create resilience one choice at a time.

Will my story help someone else someday?

Without question! Every experience shared builds community wisdom—every stumble/success adds light for those walking behind us.

Conclusion

If you've made it to this final section, I want to pause for a moment and say, from the bottom of my heart: thank you. Not just for reading, but for being the kind of person who refuses to give up hope, even when life throws you into the deep end. I wrote this book for you because I've been in the realm of where you are—watching loved ones struggle, feeling helpless, angry, and hungry for answers no one seemed willing to give.

Losing my brother to multiple myeloma, and then watching my sister and her husband face their own diagnoses, ripped my world apart. The pain, the questions, the late-night research marathons—I never imagined my life would revolve around the word "cancer." But here we are, you and me, brought together by loss, love, and the need for something more than "just wait and see" or that a four-percent survival rate "is all we can do." My hope has always been to offer facts, clarity, and—most importantly—real choices for people who want to take an active role in healing.

Let's look back for a moment at what we've covered together. You've traveled through the fascinating (and sometimes frustrating) history of cancer research. We talked about visionaries like Otto Warburg, Young Hee Ko, and Thomas Seyfried—scientists who dared to ask different questions and pursue the metabolic roots of cancer, even when the world wanted to focus only on genes.

You learned the real science behind drugs like fenbendazole and ivermectin—how they went from the vet's office to the hearts and minds of people fighting cancer. We broke down their mechanisms, dosing protocols, safety checklists, and the real, messy stories of people like Joe Tippens, who took risks when they had little left to lose.

We explored metabolic therapies—ketogenic and carnivore diets—not as fads, but as tools to shift your body's chemistry and starve cancer cells in ways that standard care ignores. You now know how to track your glucose-ketone index, plan meals, and troubleshoot along the way.

We dove into protocols like 3BP and hyperbaric oxygen therapy (HBOT)—options that may help standard treatments work better or reduce the need for harsh regimens. You've seen how these fit into a bigger, more hopeful picture of cancer care.

We didn't stop at theory. You learned how to source repurposed drugs safely, spot scams, and navigate the legal gray zones with caution and confidence. You have practical guides on how to integrate these therapies with conventional medicine, communicate with your healthcare team, and build a protocol that respects both innovation and safety.

If you take away nothing else, let it be this: you now have practical, evidence-based tools. You have checklists for safety, sourcing, and symptom tracking. You have templates to help you monitor progress, protocols to guide your choices, and communication scripts to keep your doctors in the loop. And maybe most valuable of all, you have a framework for customizing your own integrative approach—one that puts you at the center.

But let's not pretend any of this is easy. Navigating cancer outside the mainstream can be lonely, overwhelming, and scary. You face skepticism, sometimes even from the people meant to help you most. You have to dig deep—question, advocate, and stand your ground. That takes grit. It takes vulnerability. It takes a willingness to try, fail, and try again. If you've done that, or even just considered it, you're already braver than you think.

You don't have to do it all alone. One of my biggest lessons is that healing is a team sport. The best outcomes happen when you use these tools not to fight your medical team, but to join forces with them. Take your research, your tracking sheets and journals, your hopes, and your questions into the exam room. See your doctors as partners. Collaborate. Be honest about what you're trying and why—and be open to their concerns and expertise. This is how you build a treatment plan that is both safe and maximally effective. It's how you become the captain of your ship, not just a passenger.

Cancer care is always changing. New research, new therapies, new stories—there's always something on the horizon. Stay curious. Stay open. Use forums, support groups, podcasts, and patient communities to keep learning. Share what you discover, and don't be afraid to let your protocol evolve as your needs and the science shift.

But please, don't forget: health is about more than drugs, diets, or lab results. True healing means tending to your mind, heart, and spirit. Take time to breathe. Walk barefoot in the grass. Get direct sunlight. Build rituals that ground you—whether that's prayer, meditation, music, or simply sitting quietly with someone who cares. Let your faith or sense of purpose be a well you can return to, especially on the hardest days. Lean on your support network, and let others carry you when you're tired. Healing is not a solo act, and you deserve connection and compassion as much as you deserve good science.

Thank you for trusting me with your time and your story. Thank you for letting me walk with you, even if just for these pages. You are not alone—not in your fear, not in your hope, and not in your desire to live fully, no matter what cancer throws your way.

So here's my invitation—my call to action. Take the next step, whatever that looks like for you. Maybe it's trying a new protocol, reaching out to a support group, or scheduling a real, honest talk with your care team. Maybe it's simply sharing your experience with someone else, or just giving yourself credit for making it this far.

And if you have questions, feedback, or a story to share, I'd love to hear from you. Connect with a community, and help the next person who finds themselves lost and searching for hope.

To everyone reading: you are worthy of care, of clarity, and of a future shaped by your own choices. I am rooting for you—today, tomorrow, always.

Marsha

PS: I would so appreciate your taking a moment to leave an honest review, which helps others who are searching for this content more easily find it. Just scan the QR code below, or visit the link to be taken directly to the review page on Amazon.

SCAN ME

https://www.amazon.com/review/create-review/?channel=glance-detail&asin=1966942109&ie=UTF8

Resources

Tracking, Monitoring, and Planning

For structured symptom monitoring, lab tracking, and protocol planning forms, readers may enjoy using the companion workbook, *90-Day Metabolic Protocol & Monitoring Workbook: A Structured Companion to Fenbendazole & Ivermectin Protocols For Cancer*, available on Amazon as part of the *Metabolic Framework Cancer* series.

Sample COA

Sample Certificate of Analysis (COA)

Company Name: Herbal Health Laboratories
Address: 1234 Wellness Way, Springfield, OH 45501, USA
Phone: (555) 123-4567
Email: quality@herbalhealthlabs.com

1. Product Information

Field	Details
Product Name	Turmeric Root Powder (Curcuma longa)
Batch/Lot Number	TR-240815
Manufacturing Date	August 15, 2024
Expiration Date	August 15, 2026
Sample Received	August 20, 2024
COA Issued	August 22, 2024

2. Test Results

Parameter	Specification	Result	Method Used	Pass/Fail
Appearance/Color	Fine orange-yellow powder	Complies	Visual Inspection	Pass
Odor/Flavor	Earthy, characteristic	Complies	Organoleptic	Pass
Identity (Curcumin Content)	≥ 95% curcuminoids	96.2%	HPLC	Pass
Moisture Content	≤ 10%	6.8%	Loss on Drying (LOD)	Pass
Ash Content	≤ 8%	5.1%	AOAC 942.05	Pass
Microbial Limits				
Total Plate Count	< 100,000 CFU/g	12,000 CFU/g	USP <2021>	Pass
Yeast & Mold	< 1,000 CFU/g	180 CFU/g	USP <2021>	Pass
E. coli	Negative	None detected	USP <2022>	Pass
Salmonella	Negative	None detected	USP <2022>	Pass
Heavy Metals				
Lead (Pb)	< 2.0 ppm	0.4 ppm	ICP-MS	Pass
Arsenic (As)	< 1.0 ppm	0.2 ppm	ICP-MS	Pass
Cadmium (Cd)	< 0.5 ppm	0.05 ppm	ICP-MS	Pass
Mercury (Hg)	< 0.1 ppm	< 0.01 ppm	ICP-MS	Pass
Pesticide Residue	Meets USP standards	Complies	GC-MS	Pass

3. Conclusion

The above product **meets all tested specifications** and is certified to be in compliance with established quality standards.

4. Authorized By

Name: Dr. Emily Carter
Title: Quality Assurance Manager
Signature: ____________________
Date: August 22, 2024

5. Notes

- This COA applies only to the batch listed above.
- Store in a cool, dry place away from direct sunlight.
- Intended for use in dietary supplements and food products.

Patient Support Communities:

Smart Patients

Description: A broad patient-and-caregiver forum covering many illnesses, including cancer and complementary/alternative therapies.
Link: https://www.smartpatients.com

Relevant threads:

- "Has anyone tried Fenbendazole?" https://www.smartpatients.com/conversations/has-anyone-tried-fen
- "Fenbendazole + immunotherapy?? Ivermectin + …" https://www.smartpatients.com/conversations/fbz-immunotherapy-ivm Smart Patients+1
- Why it's helpful: Allows open discussion of off-label drug use, patient experiences, side-effects, and layering treatments with standard care.
- Tip: Register free, use search filters for keywords (e.g., "fenbendazole", "ivermectin"), read older posts to understand trends.

Cancer Survivors Network (CSN)

Description: A peer support network for cancer patients, survivors, caregivers, with discussion boards by cancer type and treatment topic.
Link: https://csn.cancer.org/discussion/328599/fenbendazole Cancer Survivors Network

Why it's helpful: For hearing real-world patient stories of interest in off-label drugs (e.g., "Fenbendazole" topic) and how people are experimenting, alongside their conventional care.

Tip: Browse by cancer type, look for subthreads about "alternative" or "complementary" treatments; keep in mind these posts are anecdotal.

Cancer Chat (Cancer Research UK) "Ask the Nurses" Forum

Description: Moderated by a major charity, this allows patients to ask questions including about alternative therapies; though more cautious, still useful for peer input plus nurse commentary.

Link: https://cancerchat.cancerresearchuk.org/f/ask-the-nurses/124361/fenbendazole-and-antihelmintics-in-the-treatment-of-cancer Cancer Chat

Why it's helpful: One of the more clinical-adjacent communities where off-label treatment questions (like fenbendazole) are discussed with some professional commentary.

Tip: Use this forum for balanced views, especially helpful when you want both personal stories and therapeutic caution.

Facebook Groups & Private Social Media Communities

Joe Tippens has a Facebook community that discusses his protocol. It is for patients and caregivers only. A prerequisite to joining the group is to read his blog at https://mycancerstory.rocks/the-blog/ (don't worry, it is very entertaining, and you'll need the password published there). After reading the blog, you can request to join the Facebook group at https://www.facebook.com/groups/mycancerstoryrocks.

There are also other cancer support groups on Facebook; to find those that revolve around alternative or complementary treatments, you can search for key phrases like "fenbendazole cancer support", "ivermectin cancer group", "mebendazole cancer protocol". Request to join, observe for a while, and check how moderated the group is.

Why it's helpful: Very large reach, high number of members, lots of anecdotal sharing about off-label drug use and protocols people are trying.

Joe Tippens' News Interview

Joe Tippens' interview with Koco News 5, "Edmond man says $7 drug for dogs cured his cancer," can be viewed on the news station's website: https://www.koco.com/article/edmond-man-claims-cheap-drug-for-dogs-cured-his-cancer/27276538

Reddit Sub-forums (Reddit r/cancer etc.)

Example thread: “Anyone know anyone who's tried the dog medicine (fenbendazole)?” https://www.reddit.com/r/cancer/comments/bletdz/anyone_know_anyone_whos_tried_the_dog_medicine/

Why it’s helpful: Candid, grassroots conversations. Great for seeing the emotional, family, and practical issues around off-label drug use in cancer care.

Tip: Use Reddit search with terms like “fenbendazole”, “ivermectin cancer”, “alternative cancer drugs”. Be cautious of misinformation.

Keto For Cancer Skool Group

Johnny Rockermeier’s KetoForCancer Skool group (as mentioned in Chapter 3), purports to show cancer patients how to do the Press Pulse Metabolic protocol in real life, how to implement a ketogenic diet, HBOT, supplements and glutamine inhibitors. Visit https://skool.com/ketoforcancer

For a more detailed explanation of the carnivore diet and it’s many benefits, check out my book, **Carefree Carnivore Diet for Beginners**, available on Amazon: https://a.co/d/07nVJ92W

Tippens and Jamie Duke stories: https://www.dailydot.com/news/fenbendazole-cancer/

Lizzy, a 12-year old dog diagnosed with 5 cancers: https://nfgrc.com/wp-content/uploads/2019/11/Newsletter-Fall-2019.pdf

Ivermectin and Cancer: Exploring the Evidence - CancerChoices: https://cancerchoices.org/therapy/ivermectin/

Ivermectin and Cancer: What the Data Really Shows and What Patients Need to Know First: https://www.patientpower.info/navigating-cancer/ivermectin-and-cancer-what-the-data-really-shows-and-what-patients-need-to-know-first

Interest in Ivermectin for Cancer "Has Spread Like Wildfire," Oncologists Say: https://www.oncologynewscentral.com/oncology/interest-in-ivermectin-for-cancer-has-spread-like-wildfire-oncologists-say

This site has many articles on different cancer types, including, "Early-Day Immunotherapy Improves Survival: New Data" https://www.oncologynewscentral.com/

Outcome of Ivermectin in Cancer Treatment: An Experience in Loja-Ecuador https://www.mdpi.com/2039-4403/13/1/30

Ivermectin, a potential anticancer drug derived from an antiparasitic drug – ScienceDirect: https://www.sciencedirect.com/science/article/pii/S1043661820315152

A Pinworm Medication Is Being Tested As A Potential Anti-Cancer Drug | Allison Aubrey, January 30, 20174:58 AM ET: https://www.npr.org/sections/health-shots/2017/01/30/512400204/a-pinworm-medication-is-being-tested-as-a-potential-anti-cancer-drug?utm_campaign=KHN%3A+First+Edition&utm_source=hs_email&utm_medium=email&utm_content=41652980&_hsenc=p2ANqtz-9l9EjsL9q6A0j1ZBe_lXrftmedrBoFDtmyY75Ts17oKDGr_TB27m35a0rPpFuv_3lJZr7sqBsHDUt9tVzvFv0_R3WKOQ&_hsmi=41652980

Dr. Thomas Seyfried discusses metabolic cancer therapy:

https://youtu.be/vps3toi2O5U?si=YE5crEB18IijQ0QW

Unnumbered Supporting References

The Warburg Effect: How Does it Benefit Cancer Cells? - PMC
https://pmc.ncbi.nlm.nih.gov/articles/PMC4783224/#:~:text=In%20the%201920s%2C%20Otto%20Warburg,glycolysis%20%5B1%2C%202%5D

How cancer patients get fake cancer information: From TV ...
https://pmc.ncbi.nlm.nih.gov/articles/PMC9650234/

The glucose ketone index calculator: a simple tool to ...
https://pmc.ncbi.nlm.nih.gov/articles/PMC4367849/

Ketogenic diet in cancer therapy - PMC
https://pmc.ncbi.nlm.nih.gov/articles/PMC5842847/

Should You Go on the Carnivore Diet?
https://theoncologydietitian.com/2024/09/20/should-you-go-on-the-carnivore-diet/

Cancer metabolism and dietary interventions - PMC
https://pmc.ncbi.nlm.nih.gov/articles/PMC8832959/

Fenbendazole as an Anticancer Agent? A Case Series ...
https://pmc.ncbi.nlm.nih.gov/articles/PMC12215191/

An Update on the Biologic Effects of Fenbendazole - PMC
https://pmc.ncbi.nlm.nih.gov/articles/PMC9413524/

Safety of oral administration of high doses of ivermectin by ...
https://www.sciencedirect.com/science/article/pii/S2405844020326633

Outcome of Ivermectin in Cancer Treatment: An Experience ...
https://pmc.ncbi.nlm.nih.gov/articles/PMC10054244/

Ivermectin, a potential anticancer drug derived from an ...
https://pmc.ncbi.nlm.nih.gov/articles/PMC7505114/

Mebendazole as a Candidate for Drug Repurposing in ...
https://pmc.ncbi.nlm.nih.gov/articles/PMC6769799/

Drug repurposing in oncology
https://www.thelancet.com/journals/lanonc/article/PIIS1470-2045(20)30610-0/fulltext

Drug Combination in Cancer Treatment—From Cocktails to ...
https://pmc.ncbi.nlm.nih.gov/articles/PMC7915944/

How To Identify Fake Medicines
https://www.pfizer.com/news/articles/how_to_identify_fake_medicines

Best Fenbendazole To Buy: Safe Products, Brands, And ...
https://healnavigator.com/blog/how-to-choose-the-best-fenbendazole-product/

BeSafeRx: Your Source for Online Pharmacy Information
https://www.fda.gov/drugs/buying-using-medicine-safely/besaferx-your-source-online-pharmacy-information

Don't Be Tempted to Use Expired Medicines
https://www.fda.gov/drugs/special-features/dont-be-tempted-use-expired-medicines

3 Bromopyruvate | Dayspring Live
https://www.dayspringcancerclinic.com/therapies/3-bromopyruvate

What is Integrative Oncology?

https://integrativeonc.org/what-is-integrative-oncology/

Communication About Complementary and Alternative ...
https://pmc.ncbi.nlm.nih.gov/articles/PMC10485293/

Putting Integrative Oncology Into Practice: Concepts and ...
https://pmc.ncbi.nlm.nih.gov/articles/PMC6333385/

Mebendazole or Fenbendazole: Safety and precautions
https://cancerchoices.org/therapy/mebendazole-or-fenbendazole/safety/

Cancer biomarkers: Key tools in diagnosis and treatment
https://www.abcam.com/en-us/knowledge-center/oncology/cancer-biomarkers?srsltid=AfmBOooSME2vIg2L7pgNFsPhSv6oGGxvG4Mf05grtZ9j8ZvyFhIiYNSB

Getting Covered for Alternative Medicine
https://www.fairhealthconsumer.org/insurance-basics/your-costs/getting-covered-for-alternative-medicine

Personalised Cancer Medicine Guide for Patients
https://www.esmo.org/for-patients/patient-guides/personalised-cancer-medicine

Synergy in Cancer Care: Strategies for Dietary Supplement ...
https://integrativeonc.org/synergy-in-cancer-care-strategies-for-dietary-supplement-assessment-in-patients-with-cancer/

Cancer as a metabolic disease: implications for novel ...
https://pmc.ncbi.nlm.nih.gov/articles/PMC3941741/

Alternative Cancer Treatments: The Science vs. The Hype
https://www.mskcc.org/podcasts/cancer-straight-talk/alternative-cancer-treatments-science-vs-hype

Managing Scanxiety During Your Cancer Treatment
https://www.mskcc.org/cancer-care/patient-education/managing-scanxiety-during-your-cancer-treatment

The effects of grounding (earthing) on inflammation ...
https://pmc.ncbi.nlm.nih.gov/articles/PMC4378297/

Religion, Spirituality, and Health Outcomes in Cancer
https://pmc.ncbi.nlm.nih.gov/articles/PMC4618242/

Cancer Caregiver Resources | Caregiver Guide
https://www.cancer.org/cancer/caregivers/caregiver-resource-guide.html

Steps to Find a Clinical Trial
https://www.cancer.gov/research/participate/clinical-trials-search/steps

Support and Online Communities

https://www.cancer.org/support-programs-and-services/online-communities.html

Protecting yourself from cancer scams
https://www.mountsinai.org/health-library/special-topic/protecting-yourself-from-cancer-scams

Webinars and Podcasts

https://www.accc-cancer.org/home/news-media/coronavirus-response/webinars-and-podcasts

Press-pulse: a novel therapeutic strategy for the metabolic ...
https://nutritionandmetabolism.biomedcentral.com/articles/10.1186/s12986-017-0178-2

Numbered References

---

[1] *KoDiscovery | 3-BP | Young Hee Ko | Metabolic Cancer Therapy* https://www.kodiscovery.org/

[2] *The Blog | My Cancer Story Rocks* | https://mycancerstory.rocks/the-blog/

[3] *Ivermectin: A Multifaceted Drug With a Potential Beyond ...* | https://pmc.ncbi.nlm.nih.gov/articles/PMC11008553/

[4] *What We Have Learned About Combining a Ketogenic Diet ...* PubMed Central | Daniel Sims et al | https://pmc.ncbi.nlm.nih.gov/articles/PMC10681018/

[5] *Why Everything You Know About Cancer Might Be Wrong: A Conversation with Dr. Thomas Seyfried* | June 30, 2025 |

https://www.financialsense.com/podcast/21324/why-everything-you-know-about-cancer-might-be-wrong-conversation-dr-thomas-seyfried

[6] *Isotopic Evidence for the Diets of European Neanderthals and Early Modern Humans* | Richards, M. P., and Trinkaus, E, | National Library of Medicine, PubMed Central | 11 Aug. 2009 | https://pmc.ncbi.nlm.nih.gov/articles/PMC2752538/

[7] *Targeting the Mitochondrial-Stem Cell Connection in Cancer Treatment: A Hybrid Orthomolecular Protocol* | Journal of Orthomolecular Medicine | Ilyes Baghli et al | November 3 2024 | Ilyes Baghli | https://isom.ca/article/targeting-the-mitochondrial-stem-cell-connection-in-cancer-treatment-a-hybrid-orthomolecular-protocol/?utm_source=chatgpt.com

[8] *Starving Cancer? Dr. Thomas Seyfried on Keto, Fasting & Low-Dose Chemo (Part 2)* | Ultra Life Today | December 19, 2025 Ultra Botanica Network Episode 197 | https://www.buzzsprout.com/1011325/episodes/18368310-starving-cancer-dr-thomas-seyfried-on-keto-fasting-low-dose-chemo-part-2?utm_source=chatgpt.com

[9] *A translational study "case report" on the small molecule "energy blocker" 3-bromopyruvate (3BP) as a potent anticancer agent: from bench side to bedside* | *Y. H. Ko & H. A. Verhoeven & M. J. Lee & D. J. Corbin & T. J. Vogl & P. L. Pedersen.* | 9 January 2012 | https://www.kodiscovery.org/_files/ugd/420200_1ab8aa1656674807b5e317bcb88c35d0.pdf

[10] *The ketogenic diet and hyperbaric oxygen therapy prolong survival in mice with systemic metastatic cancer* | Poff AM, Ari C, Seyfried TN, D'Agostino DP | PubMed Central | June 5 2013 | https://pmc.ncbi.nlm.nih.gov/articles/PMC3673985/

[11] *FENBENDAZOLE & ARTEMISININ* | The Common Sense MD | Performance Medicine | Dr. Tom Rogers | May 16, 2023 | https://youtu.be/9vHEYYl9JqI?si=TKuS0BBXxg3BAraZ

[12] *Case Rep Oncol | William Makis, Ilyes Baghli, Pierrick Martinez; | Fenbendazole as an Anticancer Agent? A Case Series of Self-Administration in Three Patients.* | January 1 2025; 18 (1): 856–863. https://doi.org/10.1159/000546362

[13] *Patient Journey Stories* | https://meakinmetaboliccare.com/patient-journey-stories/

[14] *Cancer Support Community* | https://www.cancersupportcommunity.org/registry

[15] *Fenbendazole and Ivermectin for Lung Cancer Success Stories: 36 Case Reports Compilation (February 2026 Edition)* | The Medical Advisor | | By Editorial Team - February 03, 2026 | https://www.onedaymd.com/2025/05/fenbendazole-ivermectin-mebendazole-lung-cancer.html

[16] *Stage 4 Cancer Remissions with Fenbendazole, Ivermectin and Mebendazole: 303 Case Reports Compilation* | (January 2026 Edition) | By Editorial Team | January 25, 2026 | https://www.onedaymd.com/2025/06/ivermectin-fenbendazole-mebendazole-stage-4-cancer.html

[17] *Fenbendazole Joe Tippens Protocol: A Step-by-Step Guide (2025)* | By Editorial Team - December 22, 2025 | The Medical Advisor | https://www.onedaymd.com/2024/04/fenbendazole-joe-tippens-protocol.html

[18] *Best Ivermectin Dosage for Humans with Cancer or Different Cancer Types (2026)* | By Editorial Team - January 20, 2026 | https://www.onedaymd.com/2024/11/ivermectin-for-cancer-treatment-dosage.html

[19] *Reducing Sensory Overload During Cancer Treatment: What Patients Can Do* | Marcia Frellick | Feb 5, 2026 |

https://www.patientpower.info/navigating-cancer/reducing-sensory-overload-during-cancer-treatment-what-patients-can-do

[20] *CancerCare* | https://www.cancercare.org/#:~:text=CancerCare%20offers%20services%20to%20help%20people%20affected,types%20of%20assistance%20we%20have%20to%20offer

[21] *Foundation For Metabolic Cancer Therapies* | https://foundationformetaboliccancertherapies.com/metabolic-theory-of-cancer/

[22] *Society For Integrative Oncology* | https://integrativeonc.org/

[23] *Metabolic Terrain Institute of Health* | https://www.mtih.org/

[24] *Association of Cancer Care Centers* | https://www.accc-cancer.org/

[25] Cancer Straight Talk Form MSK | https://www.mskcc.org/podcasts/cancer-straight-talk

[26] *The biologic effects of grounding the human body during sleep as measured by cortisol levels and subjective reporting of sleep, pain, and stress* | Maurice Ghaly, Dale Teplitz | Oct 2004 | https://pubmed.ncbi.nlm.nih.gov/15650465/#:~:text=A%20pilot%20study%20examined%20the%20effects%20of,reduced%20or%20eliminated%20in%20nearly%20all%20subjects

[27] *Pharmacy Times* | *Four States Pass Laws Allowing OTC Ivermectin, More States Pending Legislation* | Author(s)Alexandra Gerlach, Editor | July 11 2025 | https://www.pharmacytimes.com/view/four-states-pass-laws-allowing-for-otc-ivermectin-more-states-pending-legislation#:~:text=intended%20for%20animals.-,2,with%20a%20health%20care%20professional.%E2%80%9D

[28] *How to Use Telehealth for Off-Label Prescriptions Safely and Legally* | By Mike Bereza | April 5, 2025 | https://onlineprescribing.com/how-to-use-telehealth-for-off-label-prescriptions-safely-and-

legally/#:~:text=Can%20Telehealth%20Providers%20Prescribe%20Off,clinical%20justification%2C%20and%20documentation%20apply

[29] *Natural supplements for cancer patients to avoid* | reviewed under our medical and editorial policy by Daniel Kellman, ND, FABNO, Naturopathic Provider | updated on March 2, 2022 | https://www.cancercenter.com/integrative-care/naturopathic-support/natural-supplements-to-avoid

[30] *Mebendazole* | National Library of Medicine | Rahul K. Thakur; Shivani P. Patel. | In: StatPearls [Internet]. Treasure Island (FL): StatPearls Publishing; 2025 Jan. last update 2023 Jul 15 | https://www.ncbi.nlm.nih.gov/books/NBK557705/#:~:text=Mebendazole%20efficacy%20is%20observable%20from,the%20initial%20therapy%20of%20mebendazole

[31] *Fenbendazole safety and side effects* | Fenbedazole.org | https://www.fenbendazole.org/fenbendazole-information/fenbendazole-safety-and-side-effects/

[32] *Benzimidazole Adjuvant Therapy: A Review of Efficacy and Safety in Patients with Cancer* | by Jared Mouw PA-S | https://commons.und.edu/cgi/viewcontent.cgi?article=1171&context=pas-grad-papers

[33] *How Faith and Prayer Benefit the Brain* | by Gayle D. Beebe, Ph.D., President | Westmont Magazine | https://www.westmont.edu/how-faith-and-prayer-benefit-brain

Made in the USA
Monee, IL
14 September 2026

63117171R00105